PRAISE FOR DR. JUDE EZAKAKPU

"Dr. Ezekakpu is a physician with both experience and passion for educating health professional students in the unique journey and challenge of becoming well-rounded clinicians, aiming for each student to become both an astute and thoughtful interviewer, as well as a skilled and compassionate examiner. In this book, he has sought to assimilate a concise compilation of principles and guidelines that will help students to navigate this path successfully."

—Jeffrey D. Smith, M.D.
Assistant Professor of Family Medicine
Thomas F. Frist, Jr. College of Medicine

"Dr. Jude Ezekakpu's Manual of Physical Examination is a thorough reference organized in an easy and accessible format. Embedded links to examination videos complement the text and makes this manual a comprehensive single source for learning the physical exam."

—Richard Lyn-Cook, MD, MBA,MPH
Associate Professor of Internal Medicine and Pediatrics
Thomas F. Frist, Jr. College of Medicine

"Dr. Jude Ezekakpu has applied his clinical expertise and clinician educator background to write a comprehensive book about physical examination, which will be useful for students (and educators) in various medical professions. Each portion of the physical exam is described stepwise, so it can be easily followed. Photos/illustrations show the main steps. This book will be a wonderful addition to the students' textbooks, a useful tool for medical educators, and a reference for practicing physicians."

—Judy A. King, M.D., Ph.D.
Professor, Clinician Educator
Department of Integrated Medical Education
Thomas F. Frist, Jr. College of Medicine

"I highly recommend this book to assist students attain mastery of basic clinical skills. Dr. Ezekakpu has a wealth of experience teaching physical exam skills which is explained expertly in this book."

—Jill A. Forbess, MD FAAP
Assistant Professor of Pediatrics
Thomas F. Frist College of Medicine

"I highly endorse the Manual of Physical Examination by Dr. Jude Ezekakpu for anyone pursuing a career in medicine. This comprehensive guide is indispensable for mastering clinical skills and the art of physical examination, making it essential both before and during clinical rotations. I am enthusiastic about recommending this invaluable resource to all my peers and colleagues in the medical field. It is a reference that will undoubtedly benefit medical professionals for years to come."

—Loren Cobb
4th Year Medical Student
Meharry Medical College

Manual of Physical Exam by Dr. Jude Ezekakpu is an awesome book for students. It is so helpful. It's informative, up-to-date, and valuable for clinical knowledge. It has great material and is of good quality.

—Nora Ofei
4th Year Medical Student
Meharry Medical College

MANUAL OF PHYSICAL EXAMINATION

Developed for Medical students, D.O. students,
Medical and D.O. residents, Nurse practitioners,
Physician Assistants, Practicing and
Teaching physicians

DR. JUDE EZAKAKPU

www.TrueVinePublishing.org

Manual of Physical Examination
Dr. Jude Ezakapu

Published by
True Vine Publishing Co.
810 Dominican Dr. Ste. 103
Nashville, TN 37228
www.TrueVinePublishing.org

Pictures used by permission from iStock.com

Models and actors:
Jeremy Lowry M.D.
Kristen Bishop, M.D.
Jonathan Richard M.D.
Kalilah Allen-Harris

ISBN: 978-1-956469-74-5 Paperback
ISBN: 978-1-956469-75-2 eBook

Printed in the United States of American—First Printing

DEDICATION

This book is dedicated to all my mentors who took the time to mentor me and share their knowledge, insight, aptitude, and honor to benefit students and physicians.

To my lovely wife, Ijeoma; my lovely daughters, Onyi and Chichi; and my beloved sons, KC and Kamsi

All my loved friends and family who supported me in the task of writing this book.

ACKNOWLEDGMENTS

Manual of Physical Examination has been a collaboration project from the start of the book to the completion of the book. We are grateful and appreciate all of the comments, advice, and insight from all my faculty reviewers, students, and physicians who participated in the videos.

PREFACE

This is the first edition of *Manual of Physical Examination*. This book is our commitment to providing learners with information on clinical skills and simulations-based education. *Manual of Physical Examination* is based on my eleven years of teaching clinical skills and Simulation-based education in undergraduate medical education. This book represents:

- Fully reviewed materials essential for any learner who wants to perfect his clinical skills and simulation-based education.
- The book has figures that are pertinent to each organ discussed. This will assist the learners in mastering specific physical examinations.
- This book has QR Codes that lead to video guides for organ-specific and other physical exams.
- Emphasis on the concepts in the book assists learners in mastering and understanding clinical skills and simulation-based exams.
- This book is ideal for OSCE (Objective Structured Clinical Examination) preparation.

TABLE OF CONTENTS

EXAMINATION OF VITAL SIGNS

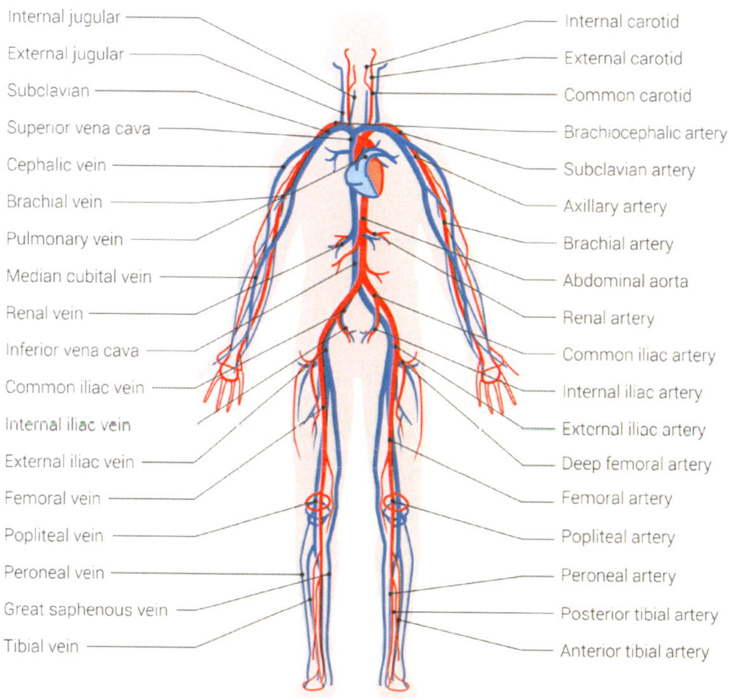

BRIEF INTRODUCTION

The value of the vital signs inform the primary care provider on how to proceed when seeing a patient. In some situations, the primary care provider re-measures the vital signs, especially when the vital signs are abnormal. Vital signs include the measurement of temperature, respiratory rate, pulse, blood pressure, and, where appropriate, blood oxygen saturation. In most situations, most patients have vital signs measured by a medical assistant, nurse, or other health assistant before being seen by their primary care provider.

GOALS

On completion of these exercises the learner should be able to:

1. Comprehend the procedures for monitoring a patient's vital signs
2. Assess the status of a patient's vital signs by performing common bedside evaluation techniques

PERFORMANCE OBJECTIVES

The learner should be able to perform the following:

1. Locate and palpate the following pulse points: carotid, brachial, radial, popliteal, posterior tibial, and dorsalis pedis
2. Asses the quantity, regularity, and volume of the radial pulse
3. Assess the blood pressure
4. Assess the temperature
5. Assess respiration

PULSE ASSESSMENT

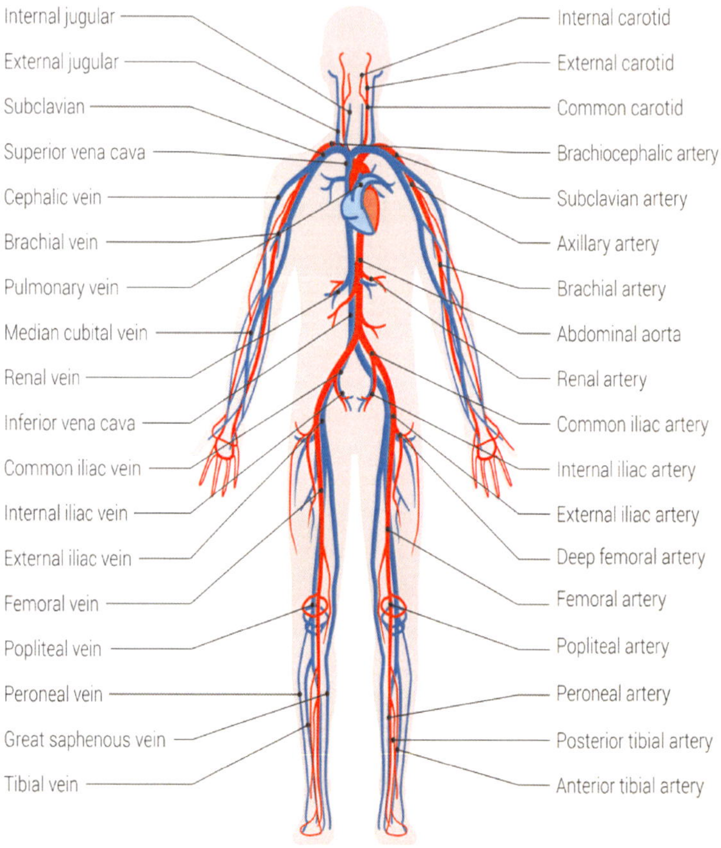

The above figure shows vascular **anatomy.**

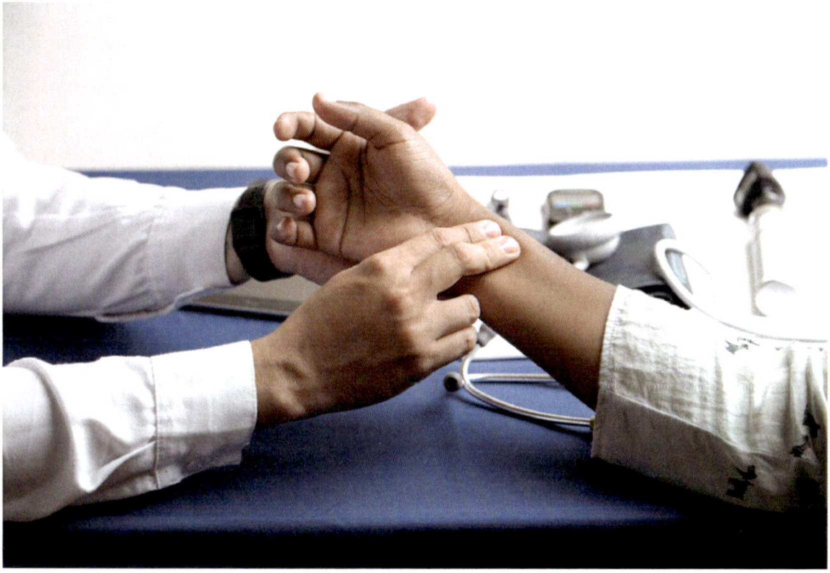

The above figures show surface anatomy and palpation of radial pulse.

1. Locate and palpate the common pulse points.
2. To correctly measure a pulse, you should use the index and middle fingers to palpate the artery. (The thumb should not be used.) Press firmly but gently, since excessive pressure can obliterate the pulse.
3. Using a watch with a second hand, measure the radial pulse for 30 seconds. Multiply this value by 2 to get the pulse rate per minute, or you can count for 1 minute. Normal rate is 60 to 100 beats per minute.
4. Regularity: Pulses can be regular, irregular, regularly-irregular. When the time between beats are consistent, the pulse has regular rhythm. When the beats are not constant the pulse is irregular. When the pulse fluctuates between the two, it is irregularly regular.
5. Volume: The pulse volume can be full or not. This is highly subjective, especially if the examiner feels that it is normal.

RESPIRATORY ASSESSMENT

Many patients will unintentionally alter their respiratory rate or pattern if they become aware that you are counting their respirations. This can be avoided if you appear to be taking their pulse while you are counting respirations.

1. Observe the chest for movement. The chest rises during inspiration and falls during expiration. A cycle of inspiration and expiration counts as one respiration.
2. Using a watch with a second hand, count your partner's respirations for 30 seconds. Multiply this value by 2 to get the patient's respiratory rate. (If the respiratory rate is irregular, you will need to measure it for a full minute.)
3. Normal range of respiratory rate for adults is 12 to 20 respirations per minute.

TEMPERATURE ASSESSMENT

Oral Temperature

1. Prepare the digital thermometer by placing a plastic sheath over the probe and turning it on.
2. Place the distal end under the tongue near the base of the frenulum.
3. Ask the patient to close their mouth. Leave the digital thermometer in until the indicator signals completion (15 to 30 seconds) by beeping.
4. The digital measurement can be read directly.
5. Rectal temperatures, which most closely reflect internal or core values, are approximately 1 degree F higher than those obtained orally.
6. Temperature is measured in either Celsius or Fahrenheit, with a fever defined as greater than 38-38.5 C or 101-101.5 F.

BLOOD PRESSURE ASSESSMENT

Most health centers and clinics use digital blood pressure machines. These machines are very sensitive and may give errors. So most clinicians prefer to use manual cuffs because of their accuracy. BP readings are in millimeters of mercury.

1. Make sure that the patient is seated comfortably with limbs uncrossed.
2. You will use a stethoscope and sphygmomanometer.
3. Palpate the brachial artery.
4. Wrap the cuff around the upper arm approximately 2 cm above the antecubital fossa. Be sure that the inflatable portion of the cuff or the area marked artery is centered over the brachial artery (see figure below).
5. Palpate the radial artery with your fingertips making sure that the valve on the bulb of the sphygmomanometer is closed; pump the bulb to inflate the cuff to temporarily occlude the artery. The point at which you no longer feel the pulse is known as the **pulse obliteration point (POP)**. Deflate the cuff and wait 15 seconds

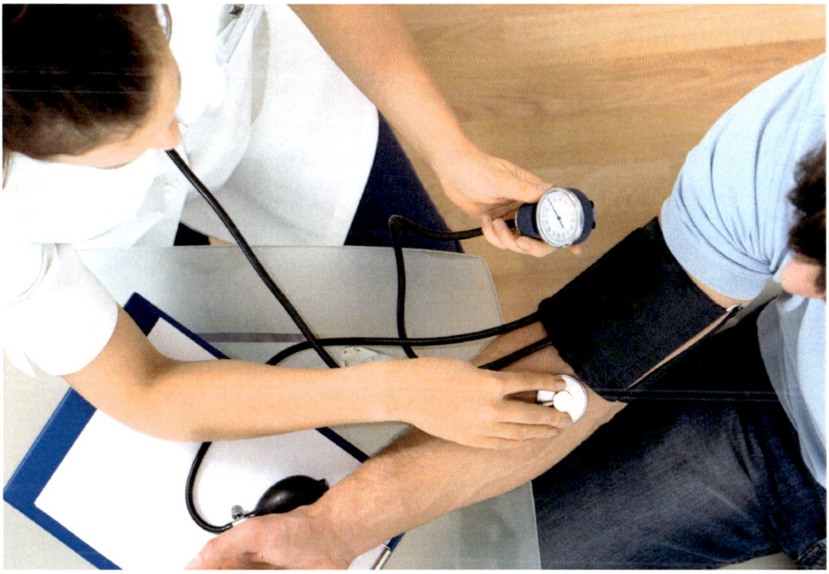

6. Re-inflate the cuff 20-30 mmHg above the pop.
7. While auscultating the antecubital fossa open the valve so that the needle on the sphygmomanometer descends slowly, no more than 3 mm/second. The point on the manometer at which you first hear a pulse return is the systolic pressure.
8. Continue to let the mercury fall. The point at which the last distinct sound is heard is the diastolic pressure.
9. The blood pressure is recorded as: systolic/diastolic.
10. Normal BP is less than 120/80 mm/Hg.

ORTHOSTATIC (A.K.A. POSTURAL) MEASUREMENTS

The concept of orthostasis is used to assess hypovolemic conditions and situations related to cardiovascular and neurologic sequelae. Patients complain of dizziness when moving from sitting to standing position.

1. Measure the heart rate and blood pressure when the patient is in the supine position.
2. Repeat the procedure after a few minutes when the patient is in a standing position.
3. Orthostasis is present when the difference in systolic blood pressure is more than 20-30 millimeters mercury when sitting to standing positions, and the difference in the diastolic blood pressure is above 10-20 millimeters mercury when sitting to standing position.

EXAMINATION OF THE THORAX & LUNGS

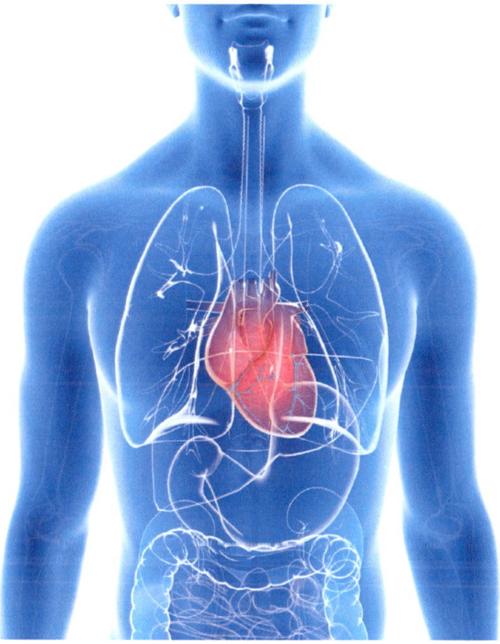

SCAN TO SEE RESPIRATORY EXAM

BRIEF INTRODUCTION

A good understanding of the lungs surface anatomy is needed for pulmonary examination. The pictures below show the surface anatomy of the lungs.

The following abbreviations are used: RUL = Right Upper Lobe; LUL = Left Upper Lobe; RML=Right Middle Lobe; RLL = Right Lower Lobe; LLL = Left Lower Lobe.

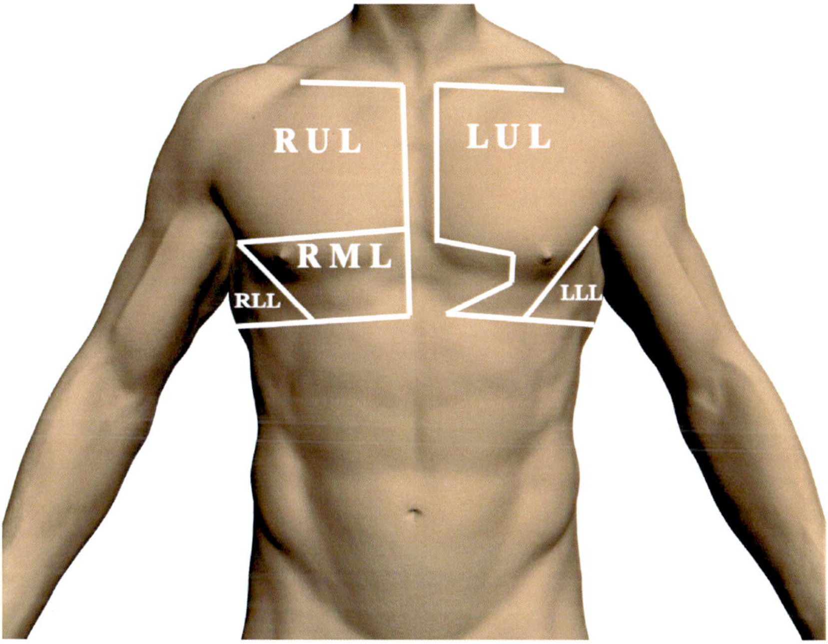

Anterior view of the Thorax

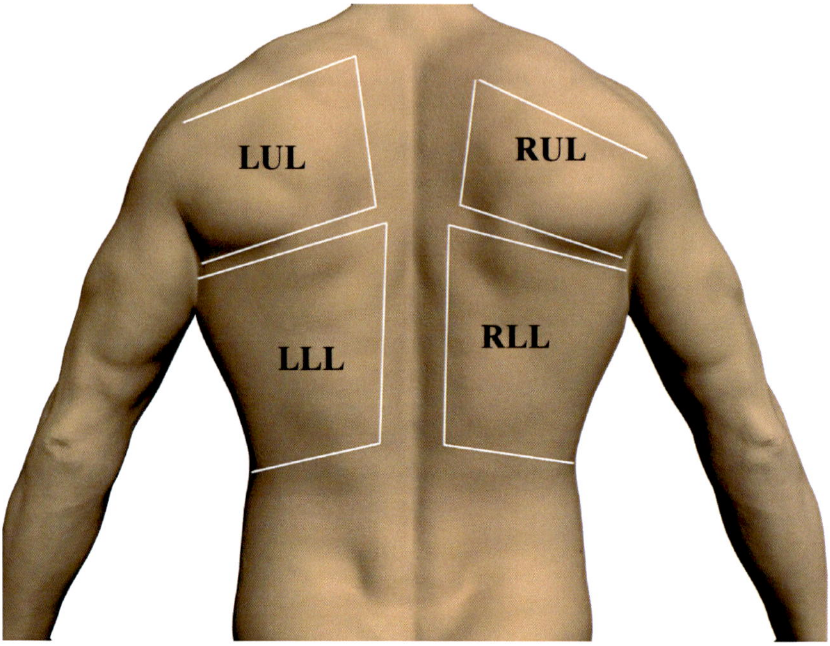

Posterior view of the thorax

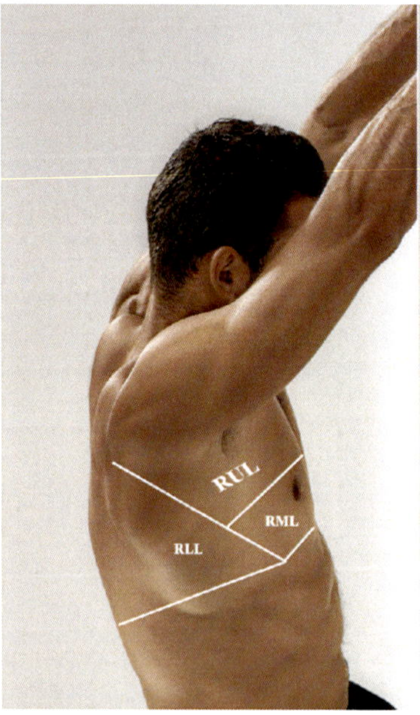

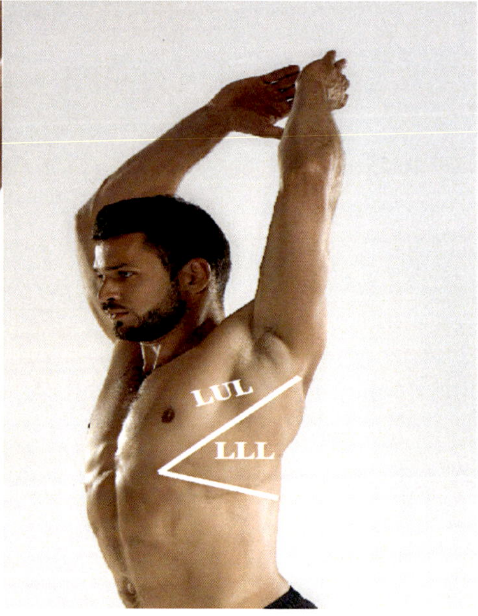

Right Lateral View

Left Lateral View

GOALS

Upon completion of these exercises, the learner should be able to:

1. Demonstrate the procedures for examining the thorax and lungs
2. Examine the thorax and lungs by performing common evaluation procedures.

PERFORMANCE OBJECTIVES

1. Identify the important landmarks in the thorax
2. Identify and know the lobes of the lungs
3. Inspection of the chest - anteriorly, posteriorly and laterally
4. Examination of the trachea
5. Palpate the lung fields bilaterally symmetrical - anteriorly, posteriorly and laterally
6. Percuss the lung fields bilaterally symmetrical - anteriorly, posteriorly and laterally
7. Auscultate the lung fields bilaterally symmetrical - anteriorly, posteriorly and laterally
8. Measure the diaphragmatic excursion
9. Check the chest excursion

GENERAL INSPECTION

1. The patient should be seated with their arms folded in their lap.
2. Stand on the right side of the patient.
3. Inspect the patient and observe for any signs of pulmonary/ respiratory distress by
    a. Facial – Anxiousness, restlessness, flushing, pursed lips, pallor and cyanosis
    b. Neck – JVD, use of accessory muscles of respiration like sternocleidomastoid and trachea deviation.
    c. Cyanosis, pallor, and clubbing
4. Chest
    a. Inspect the skin – anteriorly, laterally and posteriorly
    b. Inspect the chest configuration, kyphosis, scoliosis, barrel chest etc.
    c. Access respiratory rate, depth, pattern and note any audile breathing /sounds.
    d. Access any postural positioning

PALPATION ANTERIORLY AND LATERALLY

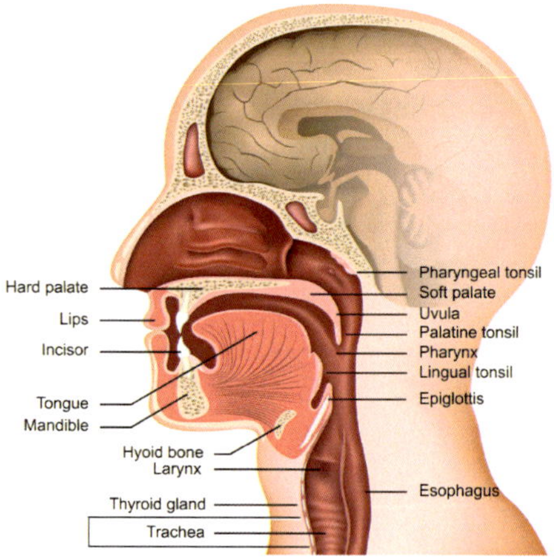

1. Trachea: Gently slip your thumb and index finger on each side of the trachea. Have the patient inspire deeply to check

for tracheal deviation. The trachea should descend slightly in the midline.

2. Chest: Palpate the chest wall bilaterally symmetrically with your both hands using your fingers anteriorly and laterally. Palpate firmly, noting any areas of tenderness.
   a. Evaluate the anterior chest excursion: Place hands flat against the patient's chest in the front with the thumbs parallel to the mid-line approximately at the 9th or 10th ribs. Move thumb inward medially tenting up a small fold of skin. Ask patient to inspire deeply and allow the thumbs to move apart observing the symmetrical movement of the thumb.
3. Tactile (vocal) Fremitus: Press firmly onto the skin with the base of the fingers or the ulnar side of the hand.
   a. Another method of evaluating tactile fremitus is to use the fingertips.
   b. Have the patient say "ninety-nine" each time you touch the anterior chest.
   c. Start at the apex of each lung working in a across and down pattern comparing each side of the thorax for symmetry of findings. Stay in the midclavicular lines (MCLs) for about 4 to 6 spots in the anterior region and 2 to 4 spots in the axillary region.

PERCUSSION OF THE CHEST ANTERIORLY AND LATERALLY

1. Begin anteriorly.
2. Percuss the apices.
3. Place a thumb over the right apex and strike the thumbnail.
4. Place finger on the left apices and strike the nail.
5. Percuss 6 to 8 key locations: Starting over the apices, move down the MCL percussing at the 1st, 2nd and 5th intercostal spaces or until dullness is reached using the across and down pattern descending in 1.5-to-2-inch steps.
6. Percuss laterally for 2 to 4 spots starting high in the midaxillary line, moving downward in 2-inch steps until dullness is reached.

AUSCULTATION OF THE CHEST ANTERIORLY AND LATERALLY

1. Ask patients to breathe in deeply through their mouths and exhale with their mouths open.
2. Auscultate with the diaphragm using the across and down pattern.
3. Auscultate 6 to 8 key locations: starting over the apices, move down the MCL listening to the 1st, 2nd, and 5th intercostal spaces during a full inspiration and expiration.
4. Auscultate laterally for about 2 to 4 spots starting high in the midaxillary line, moving down in 2-inch steps.

PALPATION OF THE CHEST POSTERIORLY

1. Palpate the posterior chest wall bilaterally symmetrically with both hands using your fingers anteriorly and laterally.
2. Palpate firmly noting any areas of tenderness.
3. Evaluate the posterior chest excursion.

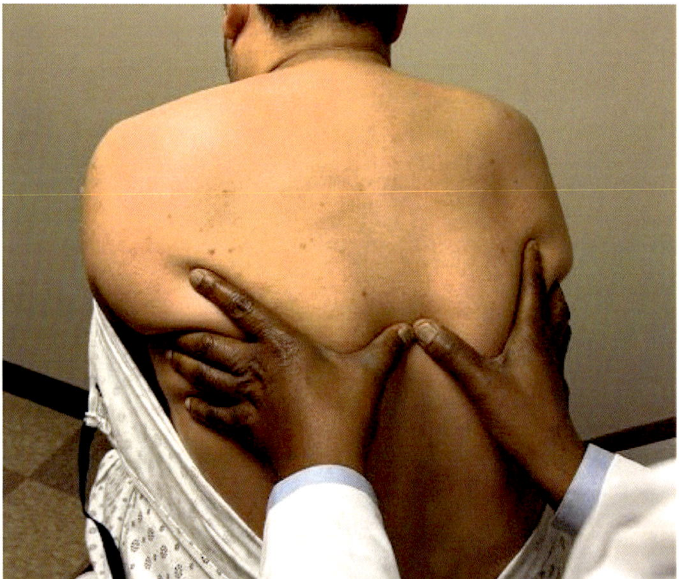

   a. Place hands flat against the patient's chest in the front with the thumbs parallel to the mid-line approximately at the 9th or 10th ribs. Move thumb inward medially tenting up a small fold of skin.

b. Ask the patient to inspire deeply and allow the thumbs to move apart observing the symmetrical movement of the thumb.

TACTILE (VOCAL FREMITUS)

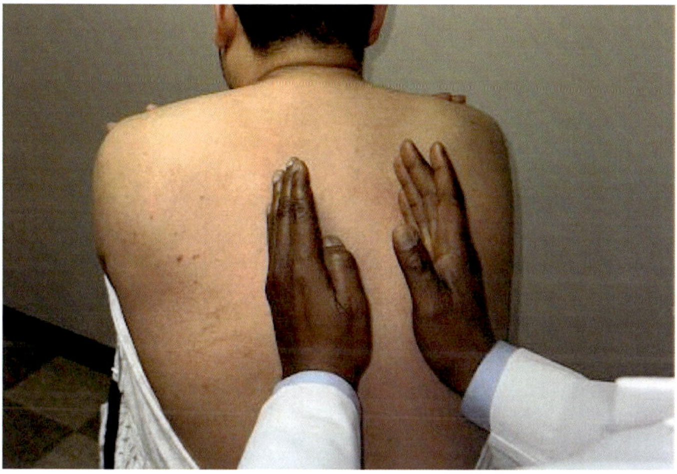

1. Press firmly onto the skin with the base of the fingers or the ulnar side of the hand. Another method of evaluating tactile fremitus is to use the fingertips.
2. Have the patient say "ninety-nine" each time you touch the posterior chest wall
3. Start at the apex of each lung working in an across and down pattern comparing each side of the thorax for symmetry of findings
4. Avoid the scapula and spinal processes.

PERCUSSION OF THE CHEST POSTERIORLY

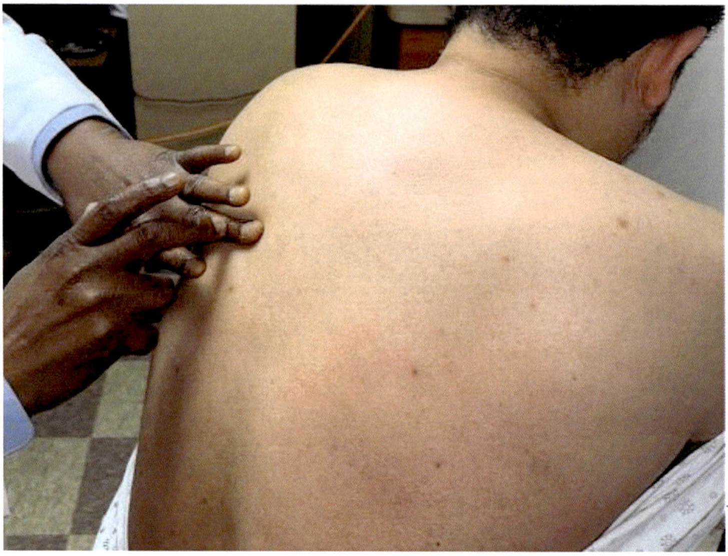

1. Percuss posterior thorax in at least 6 locations (apices, above and below the scapula).
   a. Have the patient fold their arms to retract the scapulae.
   b. Percuss the apices above each medial scapular border.
   c. Follow the medial scapular border using the across and down pattern.
      i) Under the scapulae, stay in the mid scapular line, percussing downward until resonance fades. (Normally resonance will disappear at about the 10th or 12th rib.)

DIAPHRAGMATIC EXCURSION

1. Ask the patient to exhale and hold their breath. Percuss down the scapula line until the sound changes from resonance to dullness. Mark that spot.
2. Ask the patient to inhale and hold their breath. Percuss down from the 1st mark from resonance to dullness.
3. Measure the difference between the marks. Diaphragmic motion is normally 4 to 6 cm.

AUSCULTATION OF CHEST POSTERIORLY

1. Have patient fold arms across the front of chest.
2. Ask patient to breathe in deeply through mouth and exhale with mouth open.
3. Using the diaphragm, auscultate across and down pattern.
4. Listen to at least 6 key locations bilaterally symmetrical (3 left and 3 right) beginning with the apices, and follow the medial scapular borders.

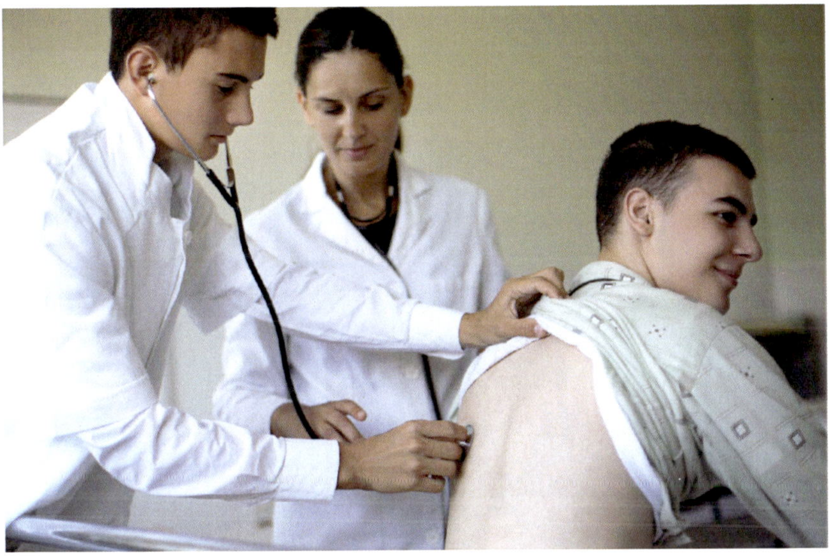

ADDITIONAL LUNG EXAMINATION TECHNIQUES

1. Wheezing: Can be accentuated by a forced expiration
2. Rales: May disappear after a few deep breaths and (or a cough)
3. Whispered pectoriloquy: Have the patient whisper "one, two, three" while listening over the suspected lung field.
4. Bronchophony: Have the patient speak, noting a change in intensity or clarity of the spoken voice over the suspected lung field (blue moon, 99).

5. Egophony: Have the patient vocalize the vowel "EEEE". It will be heard as the vowel A if the lung tissue is consolidated or compressed

EXAMINATION OF THE CARDIOVASCULAR SYSTEM

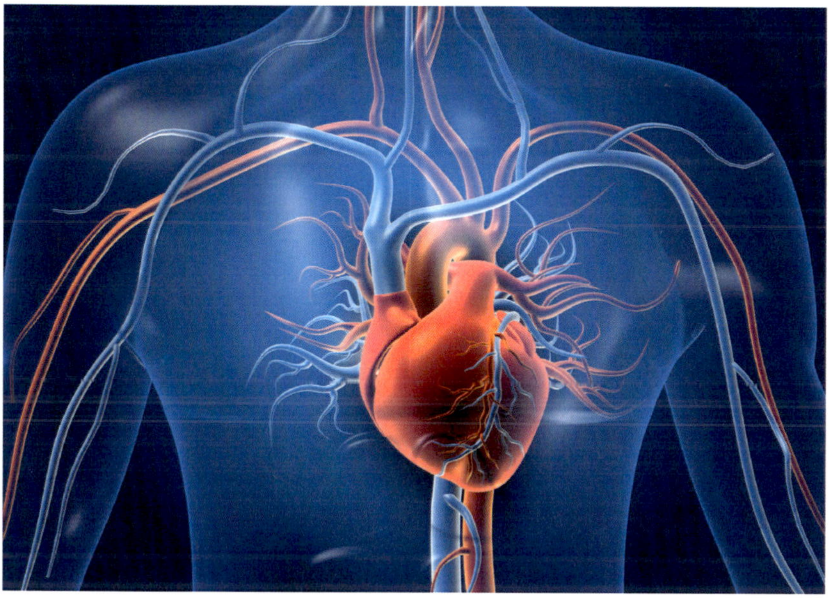

SCAN TO SEE CARDIOVASCULAR EXAM

BRIEF INTRODUCTION

The evaluation of the cardiovascular system focuses mainly on the heart but should also include an assessment of the blood vessels throughout the body (Cardio = heart, vascular = blood vessels). The major components of the cardiovascular system exam include: inspection, palpation, and, most importantly, auscultation. Conceptualize the cardiovascular by thinking through the elements involved – the heart, neck and peripheral blood vessels. In performing the cardiovascular exam, initially, the patient should rest supine with the upper body elevated 30 to 45 degrees. Most exam tables have an adjustable top. If not, use 2 or 3 pillows.

GOALS

Upon completion of these exercises the learner should be able to:

1. Demonstrate the procedures for examining the Cardiovascular System of a patient
2. Determine the jugular venous pressure (JVP/JVD)
3. Locate the point of maximal intensity (PMI)
4. Examine the carotids arteries
5. Evaluate the precordium by inspection palpation, auscultation, and understand when percussion is utilized to determine the borders and the size of the heart

PERFORMANCE OBJECTIVES

1. Inspection and measurement of the JVP/JVD
2. Inspection and palpation of the carotid artery
3. Auscultation of the carotid artery
4. Inspection and palpation of the PMI
5. Palpation over the entire precordium for other impulses or vibratory thrill
6. Auscultation of the aortic area, pulmonary area, tricuspid area and mitral area
7. Palpation of some of the peripheral pulses

EXAMINATION OF THE NECK VESSELS

Assessment Jugular Vein

The right internal jugular vein (IJ) runs between the two heads (sternal and clavicular) of the sternocleidomastoid muscle (SCM) and up in front of the ear. This muscle can be identified by asking the patient to turn their head to the left and into your hand while you provide resistance to the movement. The two heads form the sides of a small triangle, with the clavicle making up the bottom edge. You should be able to feel a shallow defect formed by the borders of these landmarks. Note that you are trying to identify impulses originating from the IJ and transmitted to the overlying skin in this area. You can't actually see the IJ. The External Jugular (EJ) runs in an oblique direction across the sternocleidomastoid and, in contrast to the IJ, can usually be directly visualized.

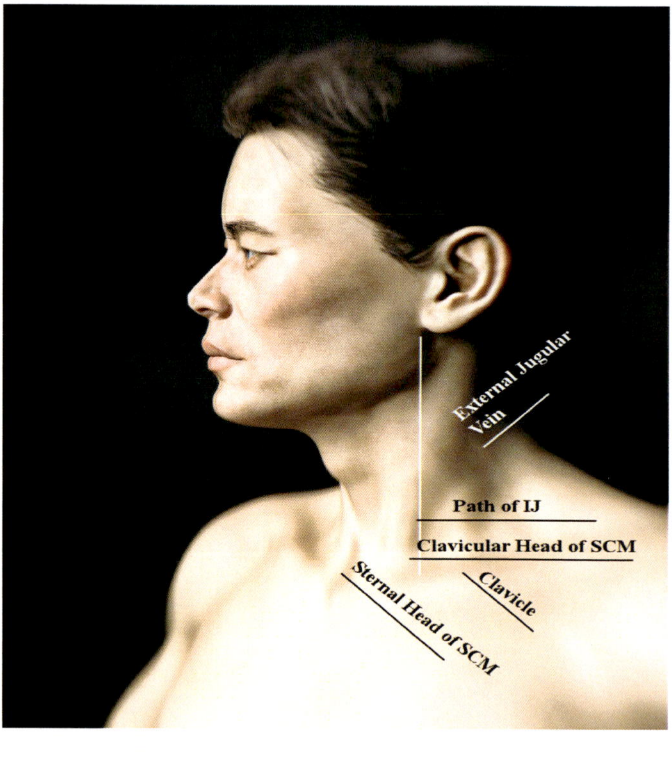

Inspection of the Jugular Vein

1. Explain to the patient what you will be doing.
2. Position patient supine with head of exam table elevated at a 30-45^{0} angle.
3. Have patient turn head contralateral to side being examined with the neck in the same plane as the thorax.
4. Locate the sternal angle, a horizontal ridge within 5 cm of the sternal notch
5. Inspect the EJ vein which appears as a slightly distended column above the right clavicle, showing a small up and down oscillation. The IJ vein located beneath the sternomastoid muscle. Pulsations transmit to the skin are often seen as a rhythmic movement at the base of the muscle.
6. Shine a pen light tangentially across the neck. This sometimes helps to accentuate the pulsations of IJ vein.
7. If you are still uncertain, apply gentle pressure to the right upper quadrant of the abdomen for 5 to 10 seconds. This elicits Hepato-Jugular Reflux which will cause blood that is within the liver (a highly vascular structure) to flow in an antegrade fashion and fill out the IJ. This, in turn, makes the transmitted pulsations more apparent. Make sure that you are looking at the correct area when you push,as the best time to detect any change in the height of the column of blood is immediately after you apply hepatic pressure.

Measurement

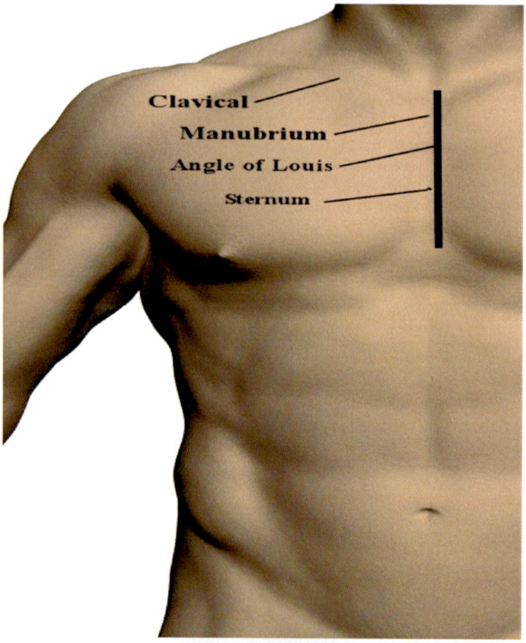

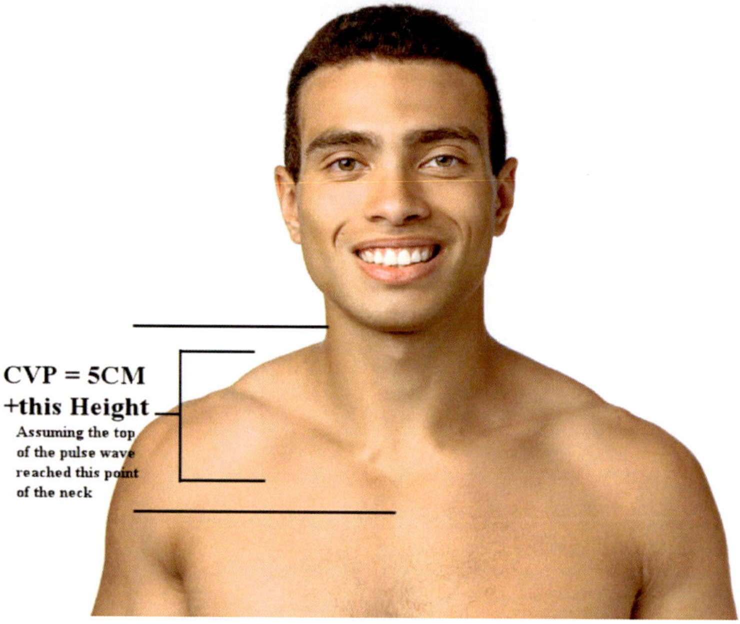

Finding the angle of Louis

Measuring CVP

1. Locate the highest level of pulsation in the IJ vein. If not visible, tangential lighting may be used to better discriminate the level of pulsation. The EJ vein may also be used when the internal JV is not appreciated.
2. If the oscillating level of distention is located above the sternal angle, hold a horizontal marker from the top of the visible oscillating level of distention over to and above the manubriosternal angle. Place the ruler vertically on the sternal angle and read to the level of the marker. As shown in figures 2 and 3.
3. Measure the vertical distance from the highest level of pulsation to the manubriosternal angle (Angle of Louis). As shown in figure 3 on the left.
4. Record the distance in centimeters.

Carotid artery

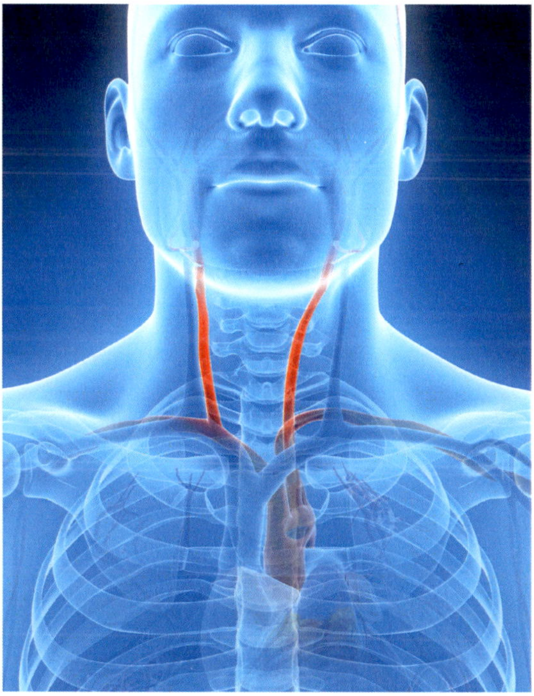

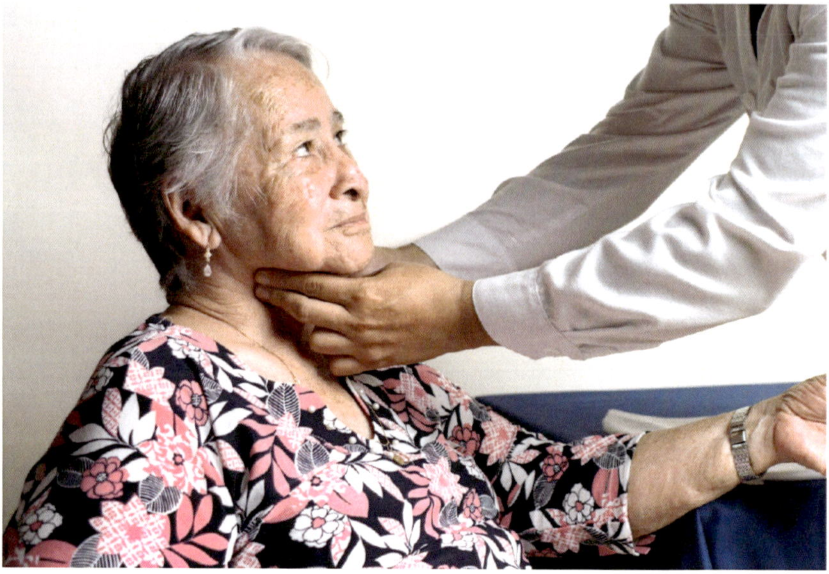

Auscultation of the carotid artery

1. Lightly place the bell of the stethoscope over each carotid artery (you may also use a diaphragm).
2. Listen while the patient holds their breath for bruits, or a transmitted murmur. Auscultate one carotid artery at a time.
3. If no bruits are appreciated, proceed to palpate the carotid artery.

Palpation of the carotid artery

1. Palpate one side at a time.
2. Place the tip of one or two fingers between the trachea and, sternomastoid muscle (as shown in figure 5 above).
3. Note rate rhythm and intensity.

PALPATION OF PERIPHERAL PULSES

1. Palpate brachial pulse by grasping the biceps brachialis muscle belly elevating it with the fingers finding the pulse. The brachial artery may be felt medially just under the belly or palpated just medial to the tendonous insertion of the biceps muscle. Stand in front of the patient and palpate both brachial arteries simultaneously.
2. Palpate the radial pulse with finger pads of the index and third finger. Note rate, rhythm, and intensity. Stand in front of the patient and palpate both radial arteries simultaneously.
3. Palpate the posterior tibial artery with slight plantar flexion of the foot. Both arteries may be evaluated simultaneously Note rate, rhythm, and intensity.
4. Palpate the dorsalis pedis artery bilaterally with some dorsiflexion of the foot. Note rate, rhythm, and intensity.
5. Also, check the fingers for capillary refill and clubbing.

EXAMINATION OF PMI

The point of Maximum Impulse (PMI) is related to contraction at the apex of the underlying left ventricle. The normal-sized and functioning ventricle will generate a penny-sized impulse that is best felt in the mid-clavicular line, roughly at the 5th intercostal space. When the ventricle becomes dilated, the PMI is displaced laterally. Palpating while the patient is in the left lateral decubitus position can make the PMI more obvious.

INSPECTION OF THE PMI

1. Place the patient in a cardiac position.
2. Stand on the right side of the patient.
3. Shine light tangential onto the left side of the chest, 5th intercostal space, mid-clavicular line.
4. Observe for movement above the apex medially.
5. Describe the location of the impulse.

Palpation of the PMI

1. Palpate the apical impulse placing the finger tops on the chest in the left 5th intercostals space (ICS), midclavicular line (MCL). The PMI is usually within 10 cm of the midsternal line and normally 2-3 cm in diameter.
2. If the PMI is not palpable, move fingertips medial or lateral in the area of the cardiac apex.
3. Describe and document the size, intensity, location, and duration.

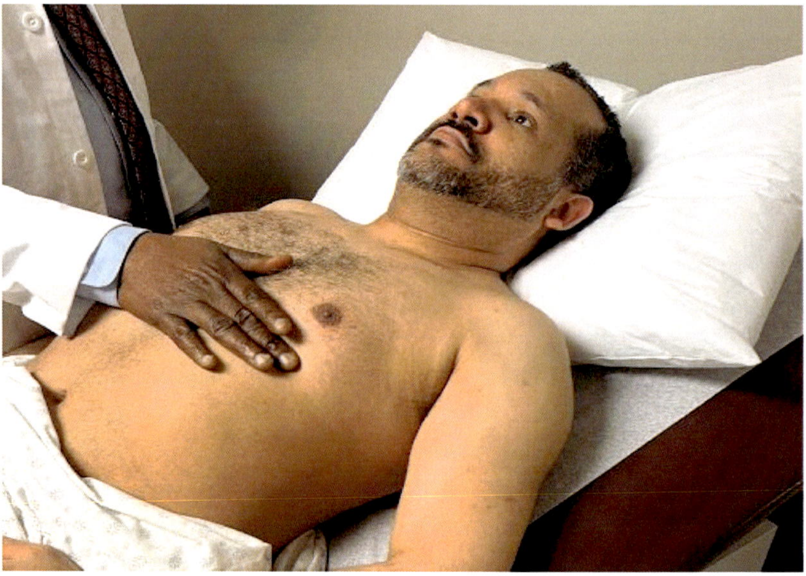

Identification of PMI in a male patient

4. Palpate the apical impulse placing the finger tops on the chest in the left 5th intercostals space (ICS), midclavicular line (MCL). The PMI is usually within 10 cm of the midsternal line and normally 2-3 cm in diameter.
5. If the PMI is not palpable, move fingertips medial or lateral in the area of the cardiac apex.
6. Describe and document the size, intensity, location, and duration.

EXAMINATION OF THE PRECORDIUM

Inspection of the Precordium

1. Place the patient in a cardiac position.
2. Inspect the precordium for color, scars, lesions, striae, lifts, chest configuration, and use of accessory muscles with respiration.

Palpation of the Precordium

1. Palpate over the entire precordium for impulses or vibratory thrills.
2. Palpate in this order: Sternoclavicular area, second right interspace, and sternal border, second left interspace and sternal border, left lower sternal border, apical area.

Auscultation of the Precordium

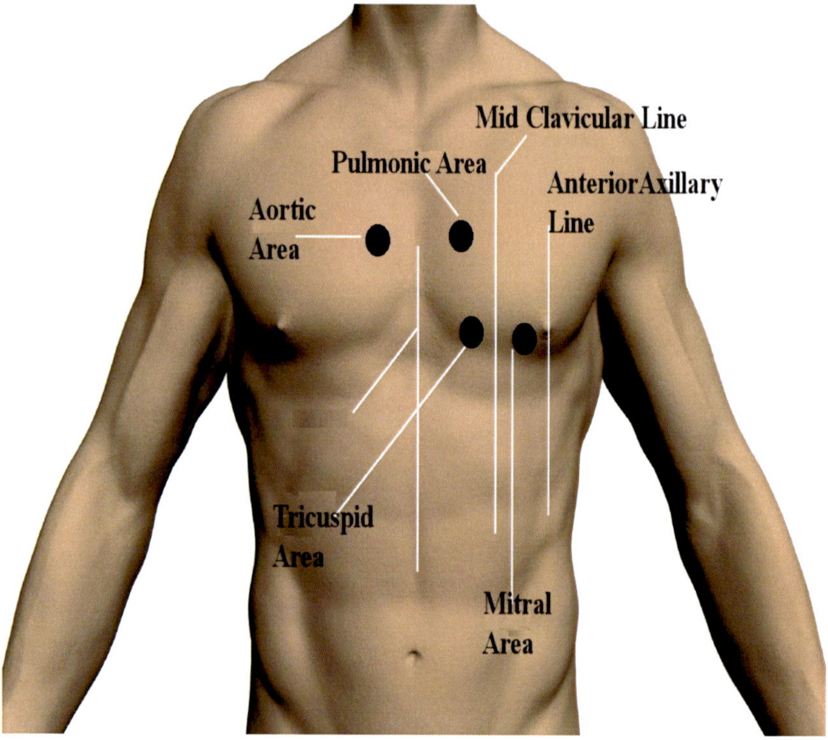

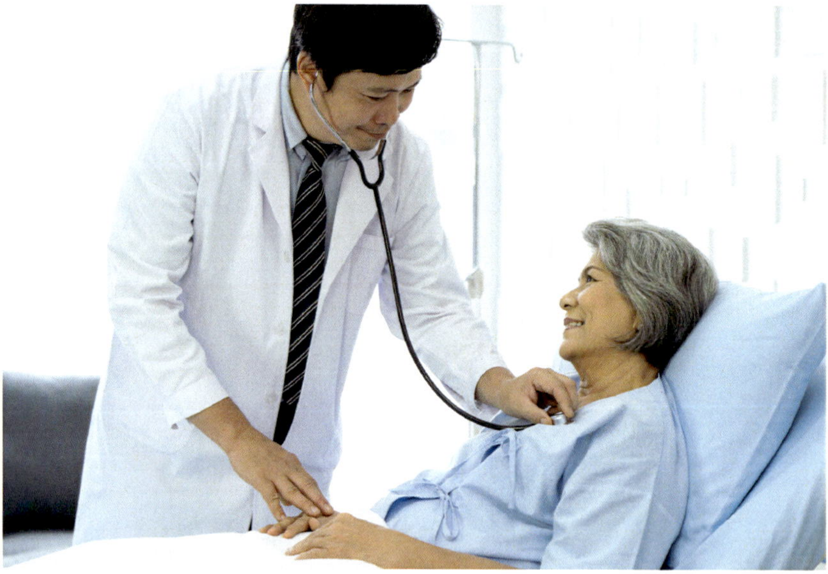

AUSCULTATION OF THE HEART

1. Place the diaphragm firmly over the apex and listen for Sl and S2.
2. Listen for rate, rhythm, intensity and splitting of Sl and S2.
3. Auscultate the Aortic, Pulmonic, Tricuspid and Mitral valve area. This should be in a Z pattern.
4. Listen attentively for extra hearts sounds and murmurs in systole and diastole.
5. Switch to the bell and listen again through all four auscultation areas, especially for low pitched murmurs and diastolic filing sounds.
6. Position patient in left lateral decubitus and listen over the apex with the bell.

EXAMINATION OF THE HEAD, EAR, NOSE AND THROAT

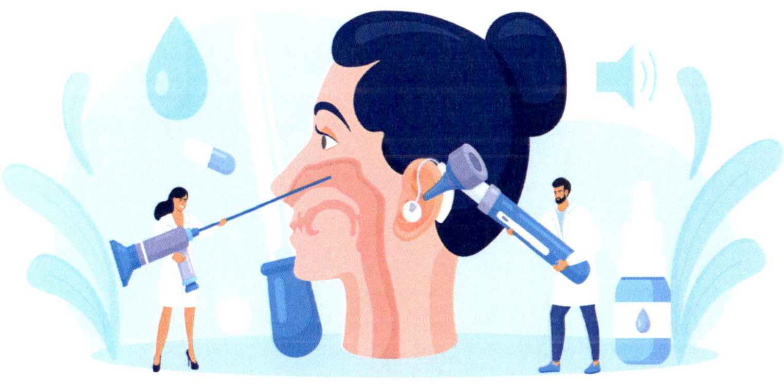

SCAN TO SEE H.E.N.T EXAM

BRIEF INTRODUCTION

In this session we will focus on the head, ear, nose, and throat examination.

GOALS

Upon completion of these exercises the student should comprehend the procedures for examining a patient's head, ears, nose and oral cavity. The student should be able to complete a physical examination of the head, ears, nose and oral cavity by performing common bedside evaluation techniques.

PERFORMANCE OBJECTIVES

The learner should be able to perform the following:

1. Inspect and palpate the head
2. Palpate lymph nodes of head and neck
3. Inspect and palpate the external ear
4. Test auditory acuity
5. Otoscopically examine the tympanic membrane
6. Examine the external and internal nose
7. Inspect and palpate the oral cavity

INSPECTION AND PALPATION OF THE HEAD

1. Position yourself directly in front of your partner and explain what you will be doing.
2. Inspect the skull and face - note any asymmetry, deformity, swelling or laceration, lesions, and proportion of the head to body mass.
3. Inspect the skin, hair, and eyes. (Neck and scalp - look out for scaly patches, skin changes.)
4. Cradle the head in your hands with your partner's head slightly flexed.

5. Palpate the skull by rolling the pads of your fingers in circular motions over the entire cranium starting from the occipital region and continuing forward.
6. Assess for contour, tenderness, masses

PALPATION OF THE LYMPH NODES

The major lymph node groups are located along with the anterior and posterior aspects of the neck and on the underside of the jaw. If the nodes are quite big, you may be able to see them bulging under the skin, particularly if the enlargement is asymmetric

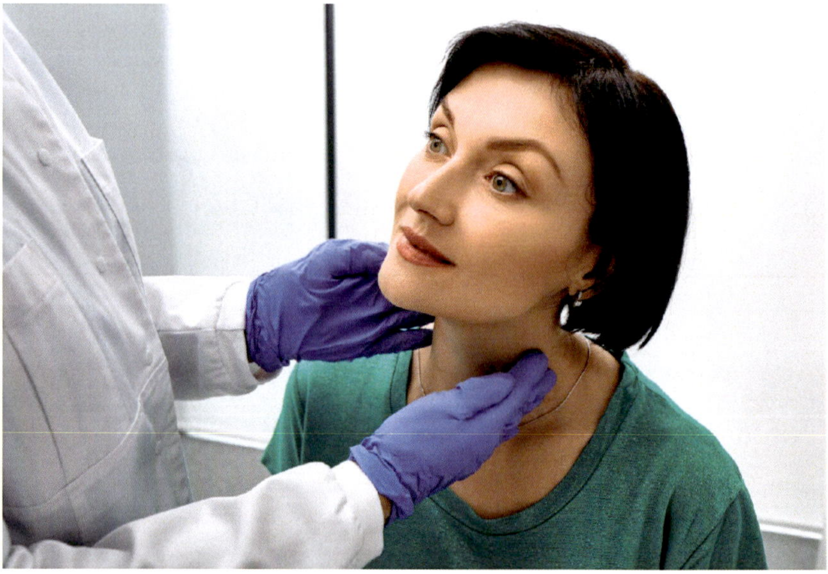

1. Palpate by using the pads of all four fingertips as these are the most sensitive parts of your hands.
2. Examine both sides of the head simultaneously, walking your fingers down the area in question while applying steady, gentle pressure. The major groups of lymph nodes are shown in the diagram.

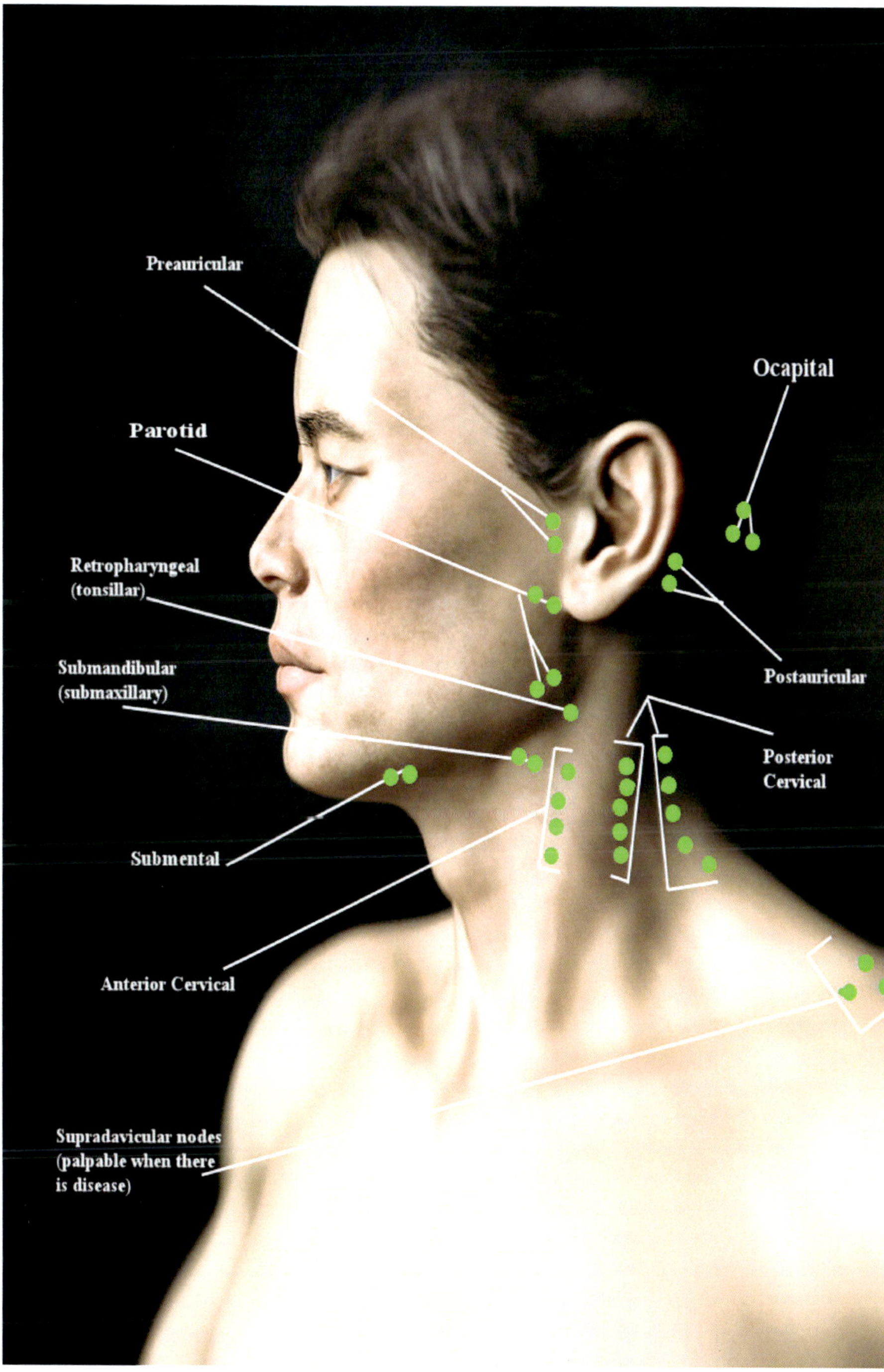
Preauricular
Ocapital
Parotid
Retropharyngeal
(tonsillar)
Postauricular
Submandibular
(submaxillary)
Posterior
Cervical
Submental
Anterior Cervical
Supradavicular nodes
(palpable when there
is disease)

EXAMINATION OF THE EAR

ANATOMY OF THE EAR

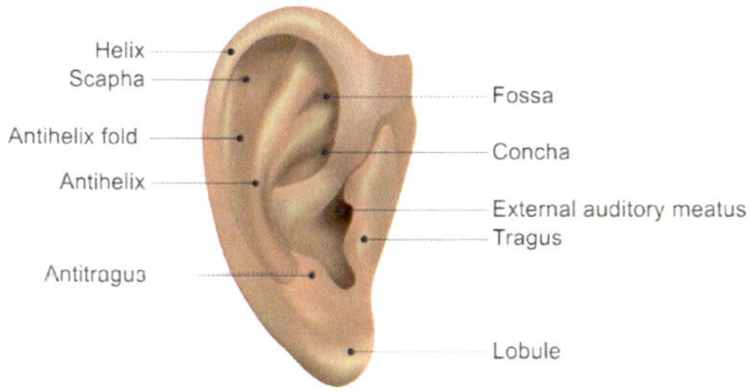

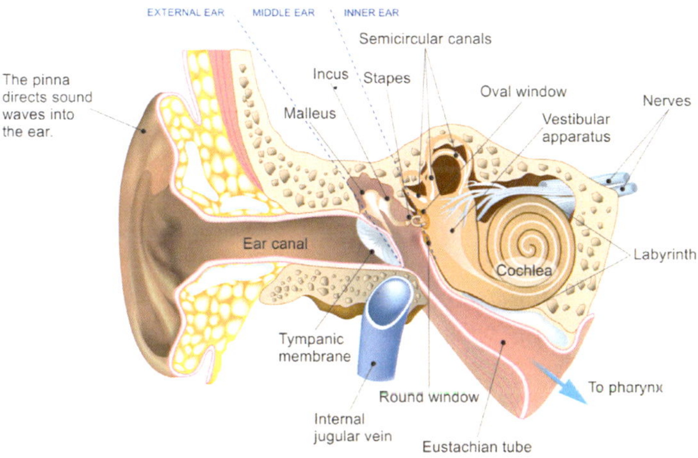

INSPECTION OF THE EAR

1. Position yourself so that your partner's ears are at your eye level.
2. Inspect the pinna for size, position, and shape.
3. Inspect for any skin lesions, deformities, nodules, or inflammation.
4. Inspect the tragus and lobe.
5. Inspect for grossly evident discharge. If the discharge is present, note color, consistency, and clarity.

Palpation of the Ear

1. Palpate the external ear and tug on it gently.
2. Assess for tenderness, swelling, or nodules.

Testing for Auditory Acuity

Gross Hearing – Whisper Test

1. Position yourself in such a manner that your mouth is not visible (to avoid lip reading).
2. Press inward on the tragus and speak softly into the opposite ear.
3. Repeat in the other ear.

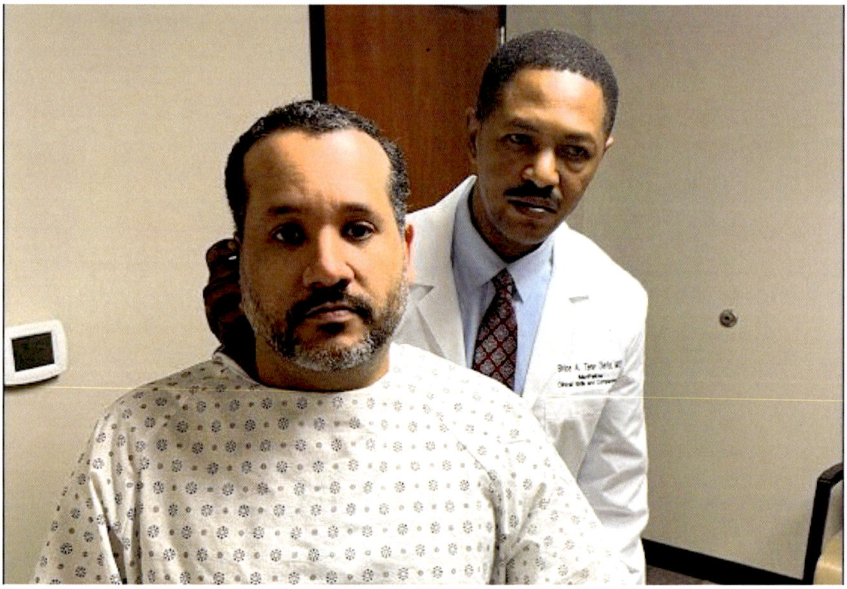

Weber Test

1. Grasp the 512 Hz tuning fork by its stem and get it to vibrate by either striking the tines against your hand or by "snapping" the ends between your thumb and middle finger.
2. Then place the stem towards the back of the patient's head, on an imaginary line equidistant from either ear. The bones

of the skull will transmit this sound to the 8th nerve, which should then be appreciated in both ears equally.

3. Remind the patient that they are trying to detect sound not the buzzing vibratory sensation from the fork. If there is a conductive deficit (e.g., wax in the external canal), the sound will be heard better in that ear. This is because impaired conduction has prevented any competing sounds from entering the ear via the normal route.
4. You can create a transient conductive hearing loss by putting a finger in one ear. Sound transmitted from the tuning fork will then be heard louder on that side. In the setting of a sensorineural abnormality (e.g., an acoustic neuroma, a tumor arising from the 8th CN), the sound will be best heard in the normal ear. If the sound is heard better in one ear it is described as lateralizing to that side. Otherwise, the Weber test is said to be mid-line.

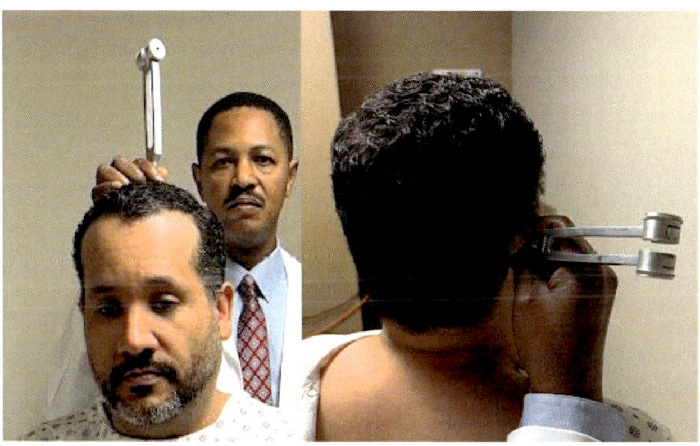

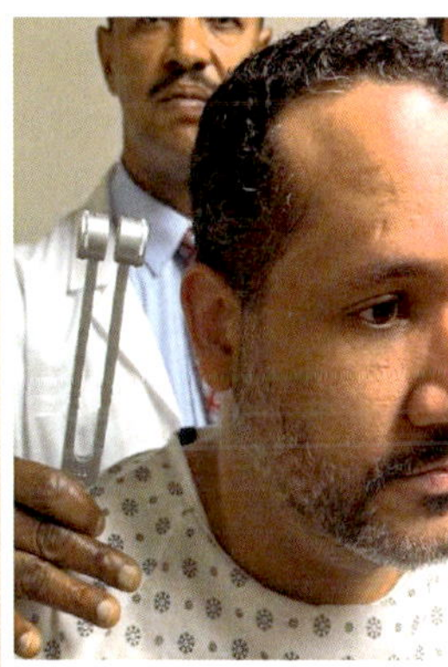

Rinne test

1. Strike the same tuning fork and place the stem on the mastoid bone, a bony prominence located just behind and below the ear. Bone conduction will allow the sound to be transmitted and appreciated.
2. Instruct the patient to let you know as soon as they can no longer hear the sound.

3. Then place the tines of the still vibrating fork right next to, but not touching, the external canal. They should again be able to hear the sound. This is because, when everything is functioning normally, the transmission of sound through air is always better than through bone. This will not be the case if there is a conductive hearing loss (e.g. fluid associated with an infection in the middle ear), which causes bone conduction to be greater than or equal to air. If there is a sensorineural abnormality (e.g. medication-induced toxicity to the 8th CN), air conduction should still be better than bone as they will both be equally affected by the deficit.

Otoscopic Examination of the Ear

1. Choose the properly sized speculum. Use the largest one possible for the best view and the least chance of hurting your partner.
2. To examine the right ear, hold the otoscope in your right hand between the thumb and the forefinger, with the handle pointing upward.
3. Pull the right pinna up, out, and back with your left hand. In a pediatric patient, the canal is straightened by pulling the pinna down and back.
4. Hold the otoscope in a speculum downward position; brace the ulnar aspect of your right hand against the side of your partner's face.
5. Inspect the external canal by gently and slowly inserting the speculum.
6. Introduce the speculum further in a downward and forward direction. Inspect the tympanic membrane.
7. Complete the same technique using your left hand and inspecting the left ear.

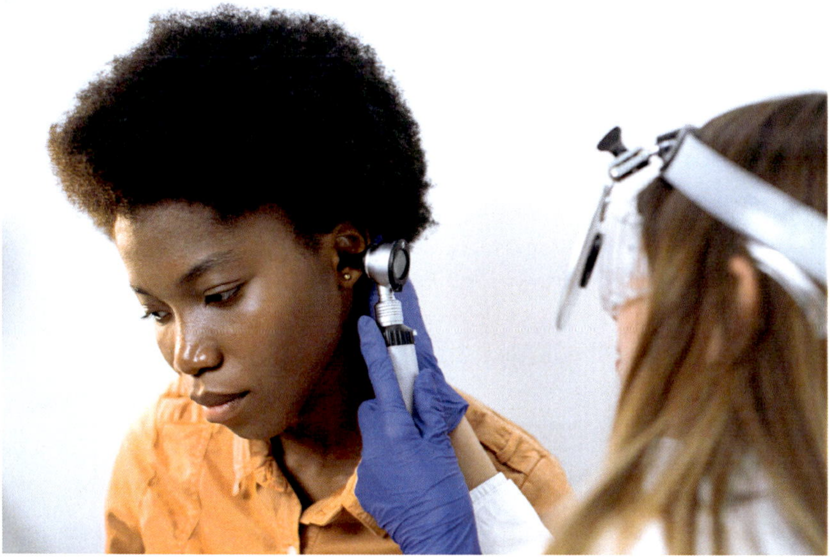

EXAMINATION OF THE NOSE

Examination of the External Nose

Inspection

1. Inspect the nose for swelling, trauma, and symmetry.
2. Inspect for skin lesions.
3. Test the patency of each nostril by gently placing your finger against one nostril at a time and asking the patient to sniff.

Palpation

1. Palpate the external nose for pain or tenderness.

Examination of the Internal Nose

1. Place a clean speculum on the otoscope head and turn the light on.
2. Ask your patient to hold his or her head back.
3. Place your non-dominant hand firmly on top of your patient's head and use your thumb to elevate the tip of their nose.
4. Slowly insert the speculum into the nostril opening.

5. Observe the mucosa color and check for lesions or ulcerations.
6. Check the septum for deviation or perforation.
7. Attempt to visualize the middle and inferior turbinate.
8. Repeat the examination for the other nostril.

EXAMINATION OF THE SINUSES

Palpation of the Frontal and Maxillary Sinus

1. Palpate over the frontal and maxillary sinuses to assess the presence of pain or tenderness
2. If there is no tenderness, gentle tap or percuss over the sinuses.

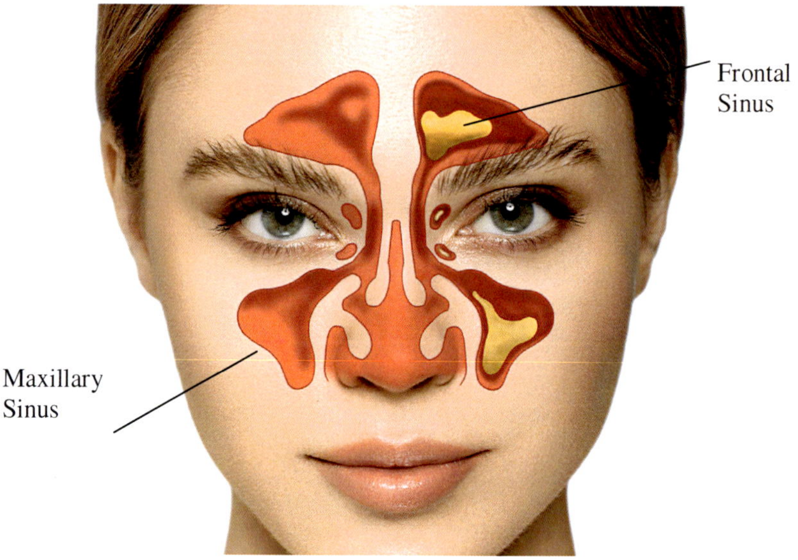

Transillumination of the Frontal Sinus

1. Darken the room.
2. Sequentially direct a very bright penlight upward in your patient's s supraorbital notches, under the medial aspect of the eyebrow.
3. Observe the glow above the eye and compare the sides.

Transillumination of maxillary sinus

1. Direct a light downward under the medial aspect of the eye.
2. Ask your patient to open his or her mouth and observe the glow in the hard palate.

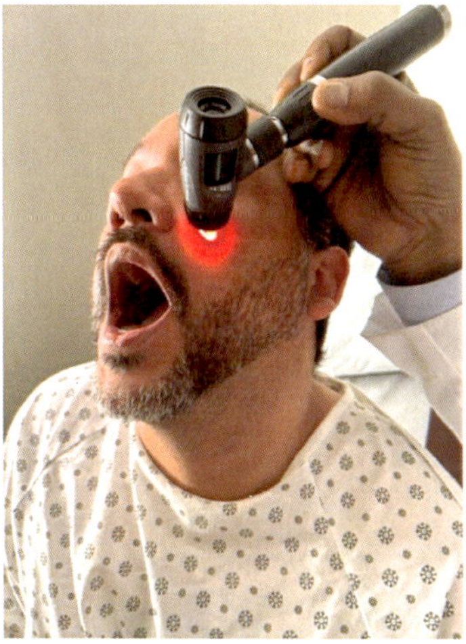

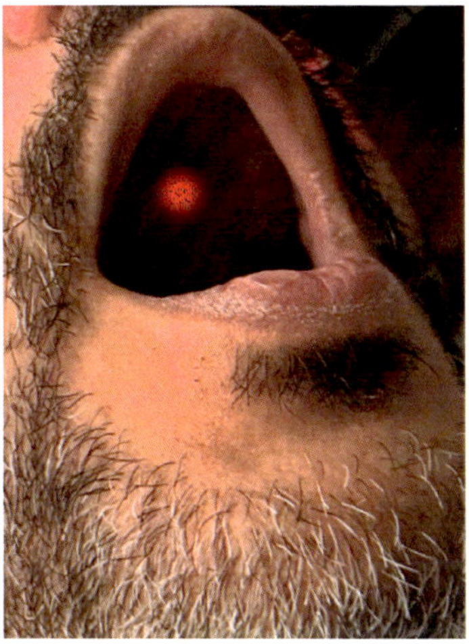

EXAMINATION OF THE MOUTH

(YOU NEED A LIGHT SOURCE FOR THIS EXAM)

1. Inspect the lips using a tongue blade.
2. Ask your patient to open his or her mouth.
3. Inspect the oral aperture with a light source (opening).
4. Inspect all the structures inside the mouth (with the dentures removed).
5. Inspect the dorsal surface of the tongue.
6. Inspect the teeth and the gums.
7. Ask your patient to place their tongue on the roof of his or her mouth to permit inspection of the undersurface and the floor of the mouth.
8. Ask your patient to relax their tongue. Using a tongue blade depress the middle third of the tongue with your non-dominant hand to inspect the uvula, tonsils, and pharynx.

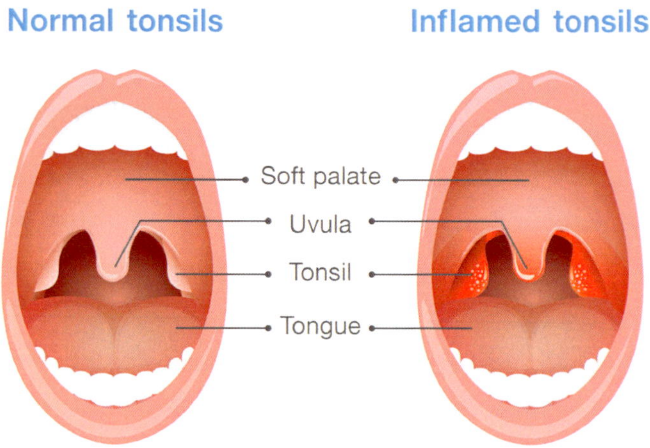

THE THYROID EXAM

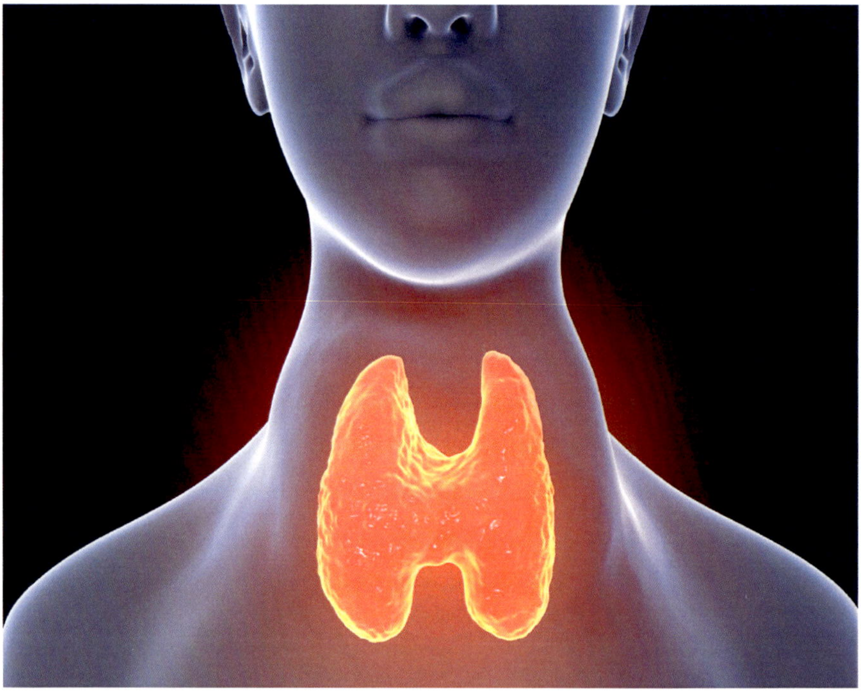

Enlarged Thyroid

Inspection

1. Standing in front of your patient, inspect the thyroid for any obvious enlargement, prominence of thyroid cartilage.
2. You may ask your patient to swallow during inspection, to see the movement of the thyroid gland.

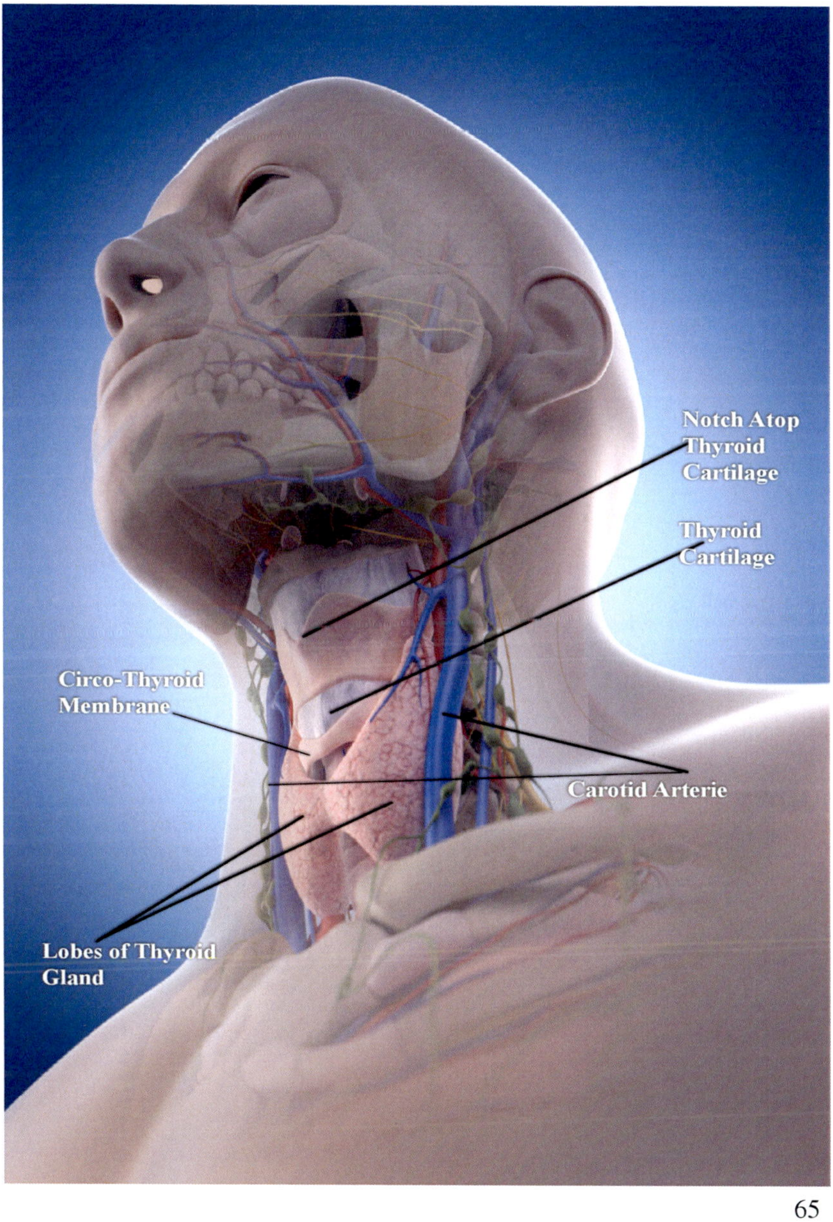

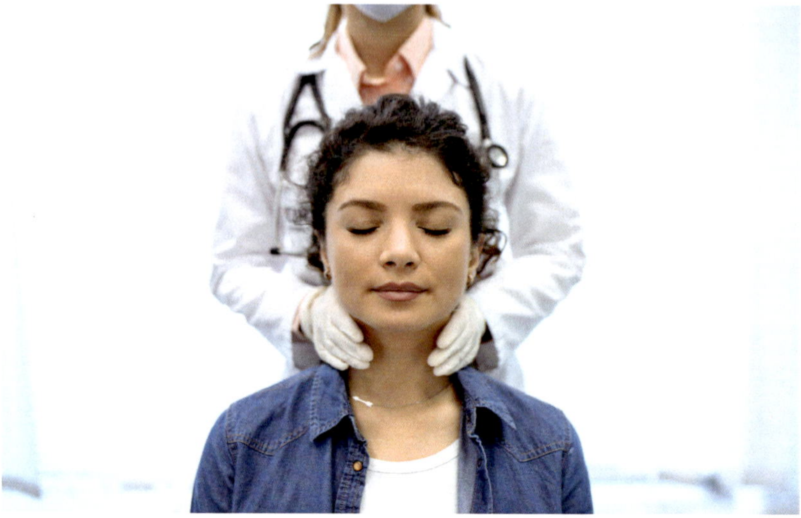

Palpation

1. Stand behind the patient and place the middle three fingers of either hand along the mid-line of the neck, just below the chin. Gently walk them down until you reach the top of the thyroid cartilage, the first firm structure with which you come into contact. Use gentle pressure, otherwise, this can be uncomfortable. The cartilage has a small notch on its top and is approximately 1.5-2 cm in length.
2. Walk down the thyroid cartilage with your fingers until you come to the horizontal groove which separates it from the cricoid cartilage (the first tracheal ring). You should be able to feel a small indentation (it barely accepts the tip of your finger) between these two structures, directly in the mid-line.
3. Continue walking down until you reach the next well-defined tracheal ring. Now slide the three fingers with both hands to either side of the rings. The thyroid gland extends from this point downwards for approximately 2-3 cm along each side. The two main lobes are connected by a small isthmus that reaches across mid-line and is almost never palpable. Apply very gentle pressure when you palpate as the normal thyroid tissue is not very prominent and easily compressible. If you're unsure or want confirmation, have the patient drink water as you palpate.

EXAMINATION OF THE EYE

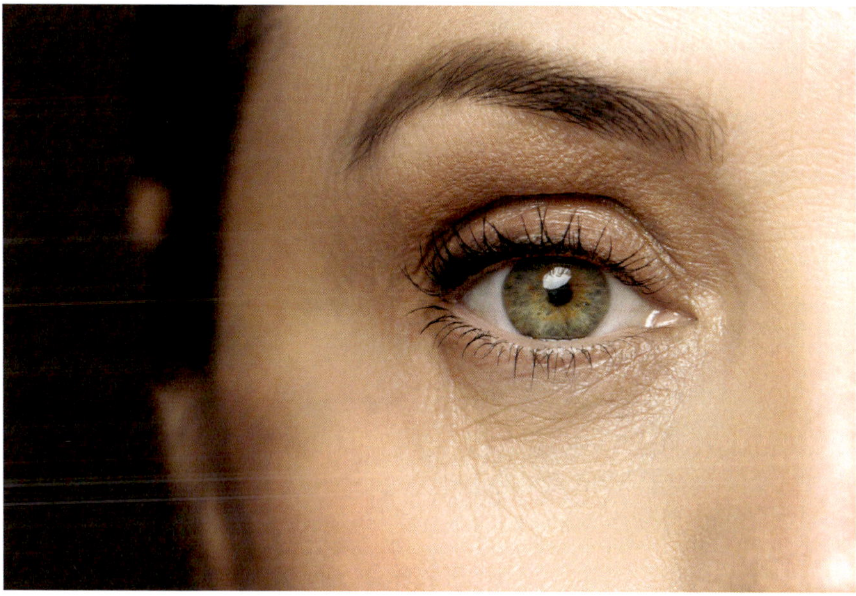

BRIEF INTRODUCTION

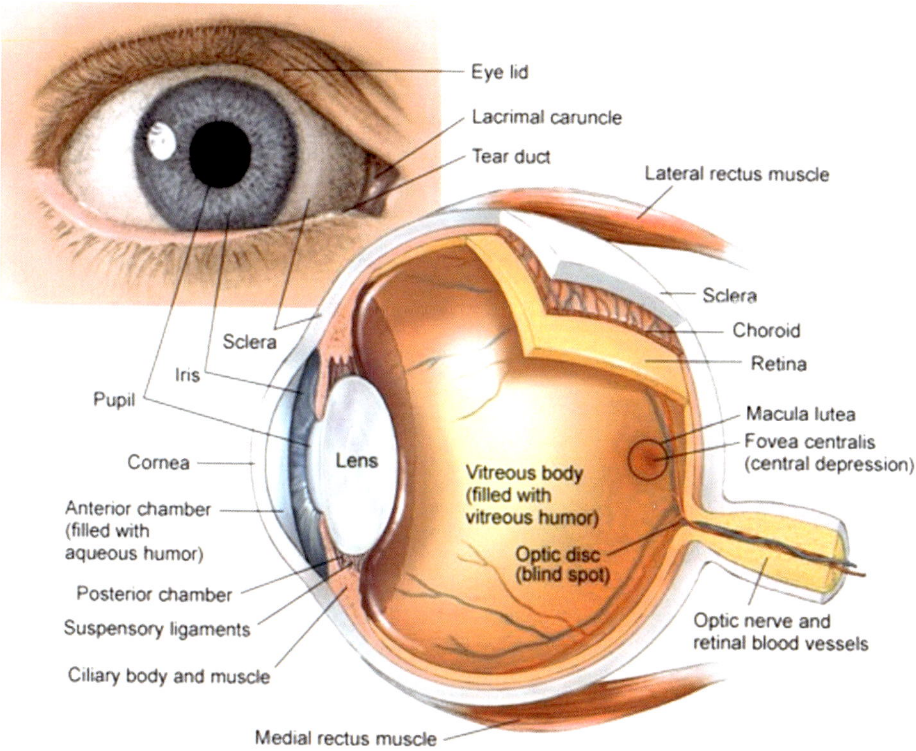

GOALS

Upon completion of these exercises, the student should comprehend the procedures for examining a patient's eyes. The student should be able to complete a physical examination of the eyes by performing common evaluation techniques.

PERFORMANCE OBJECTIVES

The student should be able to:

1. Assess visual acuity
2. Examine the external adnexa
3. Evaluate the pupillary light response
4. Test extraocular muscle function
5. Assess the visual fields by confrontation

6. Inspect the internal structures of the eye using the ophthalmoscope

ASSESSMENT OF VISUAL ACUITY

Visual acuity is expressed as a ratio. The top number is the distance at which the patient reads the chart; the bottom number is the distance at which someone with normal vision reads the same line of the chart.

E	1	20/200
F P	2	20/100
T O Z	3	20/70
L P E D	4	20/50
P E C F D	5	20/40
E D F C Z P	6	20/30
F E L O P Z D	7	20/25
D E F P O T E C	8	20/20
L E F O D P C T	9	
F D P L T C E O	10	
P E Z O L C F T D	11	

Snellen Chart

Standard Snellen chart

1. If a standard Snellen eye chart is available, your patient should stand or sit 20 feet from the chart.
2. If your patient wears eyeglasses, perform the test without the glasses and then with the glasses.
3. To assess the right eye first, have your patient cover the left eye with the palm of their left hand and ask them to read the smallest line possible.
4. If the best he/she can read is the 20/200 line, their vision in that eye is 20/200; this means that at 20 feet, they can see what a person with normal vision can see from 200 feet away.
5. If your partner from 20 feet cannot see the 20/200 line, he or she is moved closer until the letters are recognized. Change the numerator to the new distance.
6. Record the acuity for each eye.

ASSESSMENT OF EXTERNAL ADNEXA

The 4 L's in the assessment of adnexa:

1. LIDS - Inspect the eyelids. Note any evident drooping, edema, masses or plaques.
2. LASHES - Inspect distribution and pattern (in turned or epilated).
3. LYMPHATICS - Palpate the preauricular nodes and the submandibular nodes.
4. LACRIMAL - Inspect the lacrimal glands by raising the upper eye lids. Ask your patient to look down and medially.

ASSESSMENT OF THE EXTERNAL STRUCTURES

Conjunctivae

1. Inspect for signs of inflammation (injection), pigmentary changes, swelling and hemorrhage-A normal conjunctiva is pink with a small number of vessels.

Sclera

1. Inspect the sclera for nodules and color changes.
2. Normal is white to off-white (described as "muddy" in dark-skinned individuals).

Cornea

1. Inspect the cornea for clarity.

Iris

1. Inspect the iris for color, nodules, and vascularity.

Pupils

1. Normally equal in size, round and reactive to light and accommodation
2. Note: Record in medical charts as PERRLA, "Pupils Equally Round and Reactive to Light and Accommodation"

Anterior Chamber (A/C)

1. Inspect for a clear chamber. Note if filled with pus or blood.
2. Roughly estimate the depth of the anterior chamber by shining your penlight obliquely across the eye.

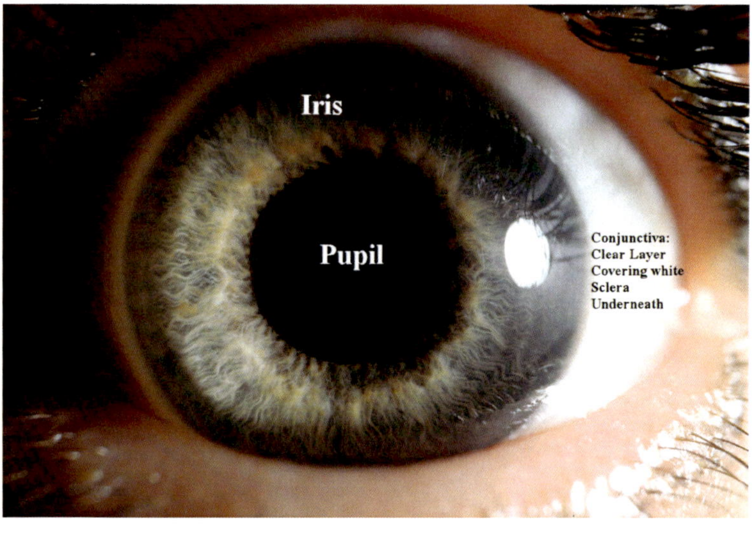

ASSESSMENT OF PUPILLARY LIGHT RESPONSE

1. Ask your patient to look in the distance.
2. Check for pupillary size.
3. Shine a bright light in your patient's eye from the side, the nose being used as a barrier.
4. Observe the direct and consensual pupillary responses.
5. Repeat the test on the other eye.
6. The **swinging light test** checks for afferent pupillary defects.
7. Ask your partner to focus on a distant target.
8. Shine your penlight in one eye, and then rapidly swing the light around the nose into the opposite eye. Both eyes should constrict directly and consensual; an eye with an afferent pupillary defect will paradoxically dilate.

ASSESSMENT OF THE EXTRA OCULAR MUSCLES OF THE EYE

Normally, the eyes move in concert (e.g., when the left eye moves left, the right eye moves left to a similar degree). The brain takes the input from each eye and puts it together to form a single image.

This coordinated movement depends on 6 extraocular muscles that insert around the eyeballs, allowing them to move in all directions. Each muscle is innervated by one of 3 Cranial Nerves (CNs): CNs 3 (Oculomotor), 4 (Trochlear) and 6 (Abducens). Movements are described as: elevation (pupil directed upwards), depression (pupil directed downwards), abduction (pupil directed laterally), adduction (pupil directed medially), extorsion (top of eye rotating away from the nose), and intorsion (top of eye rotating towards the nose).

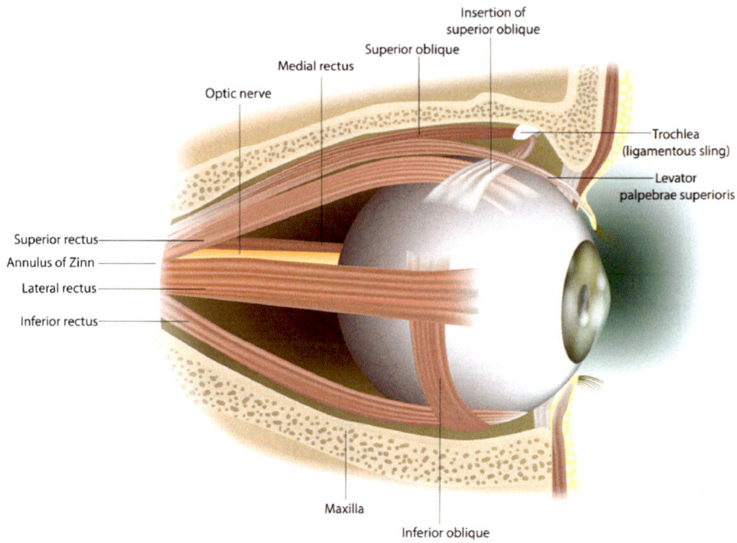
Insertion of
superior oblique
Superior oblique
Medial rectus
Optic nerve
Trochlea
(ligamentous sling)
Levator
palpebrae superioris
Superior rectus
Annulus of Zinn
Lateral rectus
Inferior rectus
Maxilla
Inferior oblique

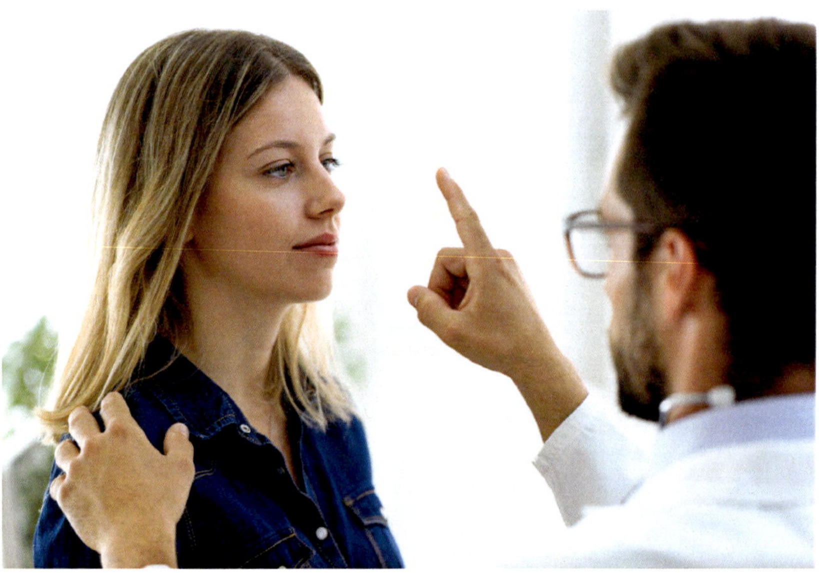

1. Stand in front of the patient.
2. Ask them to follow your finger with their eyes while keeping their head in one position
3. Using your finger, trace an imaginary rectangle in front of the patient, making sure that your finger moves far enough out and up/down so that you're able to see all appropriate eye movements (i.e. lateral and up, lateral down, medial down, medial up). Hold your finger at the lateral extremes, which can induce a few beats of nystagmus (normal).
4. At the end, bring your finger directly in towards the patient's nose. This will cause the patient to look cross-eyed and the pupils should constrict, a response referred to as accommodation.
5. Convergence: Ask your patient to focus on some distant target. Then place your finger 5 inches from the tip of their nose. Ask your partner to focus on your finger; the eyes should converge (turn inwards) and constrict.
6. Cover Test (detects tropia—deviated/crossed eye): With your partner looking at a distant target, cover one eye with a 3 x 5 in card and observe the uncovered eye for movement.
   a. Repeat on the opposite eye.
   b. A deviated eye will move to fixate on the distant point.

ASSESSMENT OF VISUAL FIELD BY CONFRONTATION

Confrontation testing is used when instruments are not available to grossly assess fields of vision:

1. Stand or sit 3 feet in front of your partner and at eye level.
2. Ask your patient to close his/her right eye; close your left eye.
3. Instruct your patient to fixate on your nose while you fixate on the patient's nose.
4. Using fingers on alternating fists compare the patient's visual fields to your own (assuming yours is normal).
   a. This can be done by asking, "How many fingers am I holding up," or

b. bringing your fingers in from the periphery and noting when your fingers come into the patient's view from 6 diagnostic positions for each eye.

OPHTHALMOSCOPIC EXAM OF THE EYE

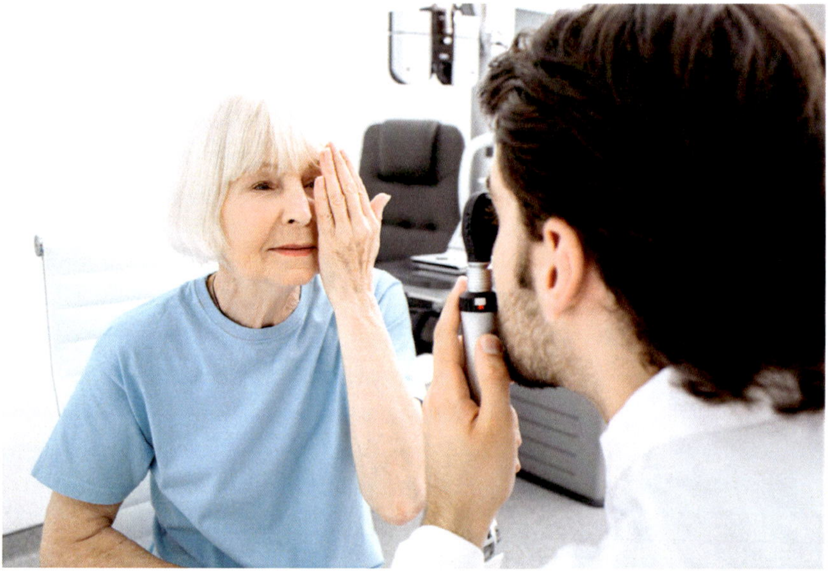

The room should be darkened as much as possible for the easiest evaluation of the retina.

Holding the Scope

1. To examine the patient's right eye, hold the scope to your right eye with your right hand (Right-to-right-to-right).
2. Your head and the ophthalmoscope should function as one unit.
3. Elevate your partner's right upper eyelid with your left thumb.
4. Start with your lens diopter set to 0 and remove your glasses if you are wearing them.
5. Focus the diopter dial with your index finger. If you are myopic (nearsighted) you will adjust your diopter dial toward the "minus" lenses (red numbers). If you are hyperopic

(farsighted) adjust your dial into the "plus" lenses (black numbers).

6. Shining the light on the pupil, approach the patient at eye level from about 15 inches away at an angle of about 20^0 lateral from center.
7. A red glow (the "red reflex") should be seen.
8. Continue moving toward your partner along the same 20^0 line and begin to see the blood vessels of the retina.
9. Move in close to your partner, bringing the hand holding the ophthalmoscope against their cheek.
10. Inspect the optic disc and vessels. By rotating the diopter wheel with the index finger, bring these structures into sharp focus.
11. After the right eye is examined, the ophthalmoscope is held in your left hand, using your left eye to examine the patient's left eye (Left-to-left- to left).

INSPECTION OF THE OPTIC DISK

1. Determine margins, color, and cup-to-disc ratio.
2. The cup is the portion of the disc that is central, lighter in color, and penetrated by the retinal vessels.
3. The normal cup-to-disc ratio varies from 0.1 to 0.5.
4. You should check the cup-to-disc ratio in both eyes for symmetry.

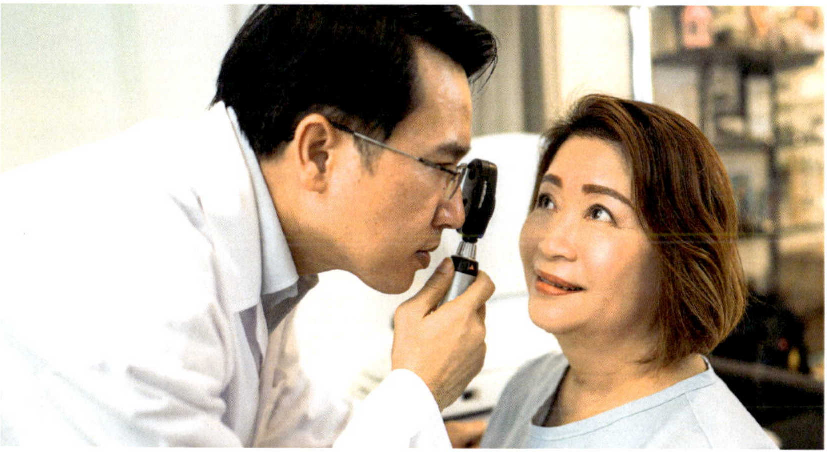

INSPECTION OF RETINAL VESSELS

1. Follow the vessels in all four directions choosing one branch at a time - superior temporal, superior nasal, inferior nasal, and inferior temporal.
2. The arteries are to 2/3 to 4/5 the size of the veins and have a prominent light reflex.

INSPECTION OF THE MACULA

1. Keep the ophthalmoscope level with the disc and look temporally about 2 – disc diameters to view the macula. The macula is a vascular area with a pinpoint reflective center, the fovea.
2. Direct your partner to look directly into the light to view the fovea.

NEUROLOGICAL AND MINI-MENTAL STATUS EXAMINATION

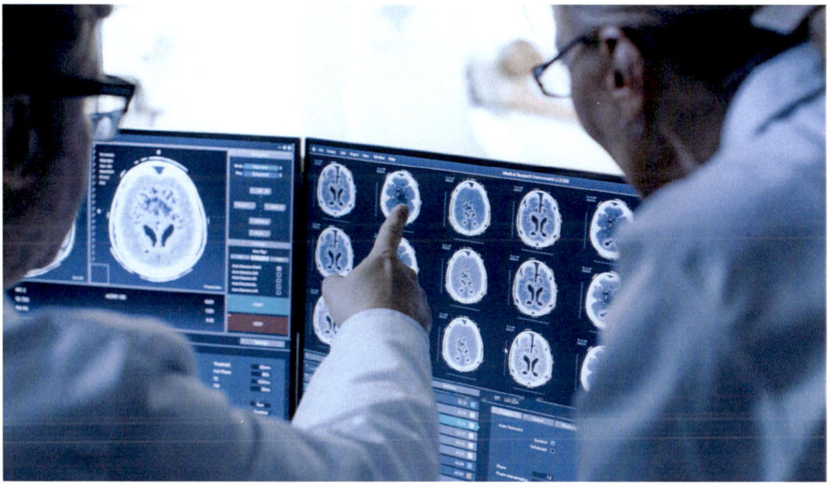

SCAN TO SEE MINI MENTAL EXAM

SCAN TO SEE CENTRAL NERVOUS SYSTEM

BRIEF INTRODUCTION

The major areas of the exam, covering the most testable components of the neurological system, include:

1. Mental status testing
2. Cranial Nerves
3. Muscle strength, tone and bulk
4. Reflexes
5. Coordination
6. Sensory Function
7. Gait

GOALS

Upon completion of this exercise, the student should comprehend the principles and procedures for conducting a basic neurological examination. The student should also understand the purpose and administration of the Mini-Mental Status Exam (MMSE).

PERFORMANCE OBJECTIVES

The student should be able to perform the following:

1. Identify and apply the components of the MMSE
2. Demonstrate knowledge of the basic parts of a neurologic evaluation
3. Demonstrate knowledge of the cranial nerve functions
4. Perform a basic motor and sensory evaluation
5. Perform cerebellar testing
6. Test stretch, superficial and pathologic reflexes
7. Observe the gait

1. MINI-MENTAL STATE

One point for each answer Date:			
ORIENTATION Year Season Month Date Time Country Town District Hospital Ward / Floor	 ___/ 5 ___/ 5	 ___/ 5 ___/ 5	 ___/ 5 ___/ 5
REGISTRATION Examiner names three objects (e.g. apple, table, penny) and asks the patient to repeat (1 point for each correct. THEN the patient learns the 3 names repeating until correct).	___/3	___/3	___/3
ATTENTION AND CALCULATION Subtract 7 from 100, then repeat from the result. Continue five times: 100, 93, 86, 79, 72, 65 (Alternative: spell "WORLD" backwards: DLROW).	___/ 5	___/ 5	___/ 5
Immediate Recall Ask for the names of the three objects learned earlier. **Past Recall** Ask questions that you can verify like Who was the president before Donald Trump? Who is the President after Donald Trump? Who is the current president?	___/3	___/3	___/3
LANGUAGE Name two objects (e.g. pen, watch). Repeat "No ifs, ands, or buts".	___/2 ___/1 ___/3 ___/1 ___/1	___/2 ___/1 ___/3 ___/1 ___/1	___/2 ___/1 ___/3 ___/1 ___/1
COPYING Ask the patient to copy a pair of intersecting pentagons	___/1	___/ 1	___/1
Total	___/ 30	___/ 30	___/ 30

EXAMINATION (MMSE)

Give a three-stage command. Score 1 for each stage. (e.g. "Place index finger of right hand on your nose and then on your left ear").	___/3	___/3	___/3
Ask the patient to read and obey a written command on a piece of paper. The written instruction is: "Close your eyes".	___/1	___/1	___/1
Ask the patient to write a sentence. Score 1 if it is sensible and has a subject and a verb.	___/1	___/1	___/1

COPYING: Ask the patient to copy a pair of intersecting pentagons

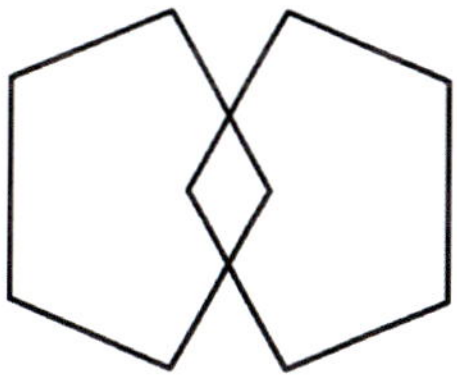

MMSE SCORING

24-30: no cognitive impairment
18-23: mild cognitive impairment
0-17: severe cognitive impairment

SUMMARY OF MINI MENTAL EXAM - MINIMAL REQUIREMENT

1. **Orientation in time, place and person** – who am I? Where are you? Is it morning, afternoon, or evening?
2. **Immediate memory** – name three things and ask the patient to remember those three things at the end of exam.

3. **Past memory** – ask the patient memories in the past that you can verify like the names of former presidents.
4. **Subtract 5 from 100** counting down. Stop the patient when he/she gets to 80.
5. Spell world backwards.

CRANIAL NERVE EXAMINATION

1. Introduce yourself to the patient and explain what you will be doing.
2. Position yourself directly in front of the patient.

CN I OLFACTORY NERVE:

1. Tell the patient that you are going to test their ability to smell.
2. Ask the patient to close their eyes and to close one nostril with their finger.
3. Wave a mild, non-irritating substance (coffee, mint, a stick of gum, etc.) in front of the open nostril and instruct the patient to sniff and identify the test substance.
4. Test another nostril with a different smell.
5. If the patient is unable to smell or has a congested nasal passage, ask the patient if they have had any recent change in their sense of smell.

CN II OPTIC NERVE

1. Perform the visual acuity exam as previously practiced.
2. Perform the visual fields as previously described.
3. Perform the pupillary light reflex as previously described.

CN III OCULOMOTOR NERVE, CN IV TROCHLEAR NERVE, CN VI ABDUCENS NERVE

1. Pupillary light reflex: Dim the room lights. Ask the patient to fixate on a distant object. Observe the direct (ipsilateral) and

consensual (contralateral) responses while shining a light in one of the patient's eyes and then the other. Do the swing test after you check each pupil.

2. Near reflex: Ask the patient to focus on the wall behind you. Place a pencil approximately 5 inches away from the patient and ask them to focus on the pencil.
3. Cover test: Instruct the patient to look at a distant object. Cover one eye with a 3 x 5 in card. Observe the uncovered eye. If it moves to take up fixation of the distant point, the eye was not straight before the other eye was covered. If the eye did not move, it was straight. Repeat test on the other eye.
4. Cardinal positions of gaze: Hold the patient's chin steady with right hand and ask the patient to follow your left index finger about 10 inches away from patient's nose

CN V TRIGEMINAL NERVE:

1. Corneal reflex CNV and CNVII: Using a cotton tip applicator that is pulled into a very thin strand, stabilize the patient's head and ask the patient to look to the right as the cotton tip is brought from the left to gently touch the cornea. Lids should close bilaterally. (Note that we do not perform these skills on a standardized patient.)
2. The sensory portion of CNV: Ask the patient to close their eyes. Lightly touch the patient's face with a cotton tip. Have the patient respond when a touch is felt. The test is performed on the cheeks and jaw testing all three divisions of the nerve on each side of the face. Repeat the procedure using a sharp object.
3. Motor function of CNV: Have the patient bite down or clench their teeth while you palpate the masseter and temporalis muscles bilaterally.

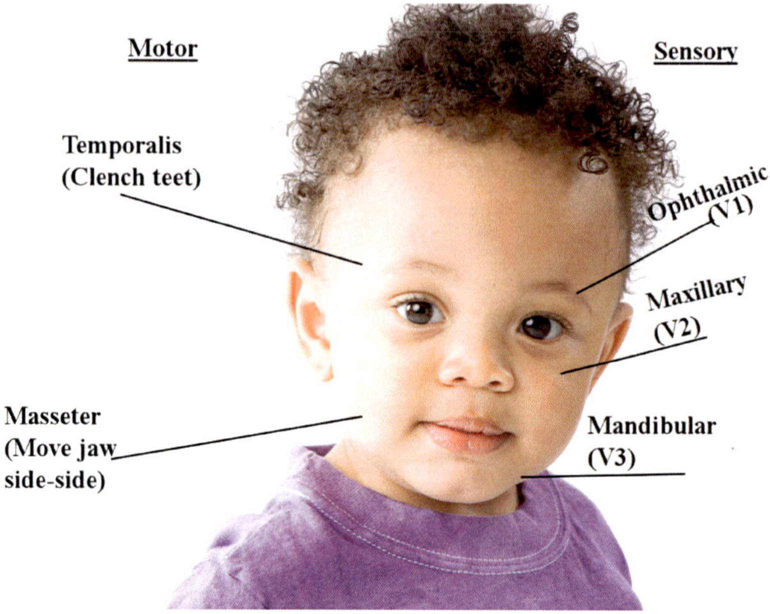

CN VII FACIAL NERVE

1. Ask the patient to smile and observe their face for asymmetry.
2. Ask the patient to puff out their cheeks against your resistance.
3. Ask the patient to raise their eyebrows and to frown.
4. Ask the patient to close their eyes tightly while you try to open them, one at a time.
5. You should instruct the patient to keep their eyes closed as tightly as possible.

CN VIII VESTIBULOCOCHLEAR

1. Perform the Rinne and Weber test as previously explained.

CN IX GLOSSOPHARYNGEAL NERVE:

1. Using an applicator stick or tongue blade, touch the posterior third of the tongue, soft palate, or the posterior pharyngeal

wall. At that point, you should elicit a gag reflex. (Note: we do not perform gag reflex on a standardized patient)

2. At this time, you may also tell your patient to open their mouth wide and say, "ah... ah," while looking for the symmetric elevation of the soft palate. The uvula should remain in the midline. This demonstrates the function of cranial nerves IX and X. Taste sensation of the posterior third of the tongue is not routinely tested.

CN X VAGUS NERVE

1. This examination is done along with the examination of CN IX.

CN XI SPINAL ACCESSORY NERVE

1. Ask the patient to turn their head left, and then right, against resistance applied to the side of the chin.
2. Inspect the sternomastoid and trapezius muscles for equal size.
3. Ask the patient to shrug both shoulders against your downward resistance.

CN XII HYPOGLOSSAL NERVE:

1. Ask the patient to open their mouth and stick out their tongue inspecting for midline position.
2. Ask the patient to move the tongue side-by-side while sticking them out

EXAMINATION OF THE MOTOR FUNCTION

UPPER EXTREMITIES

1. Inspect the upper extremities for symmetry.
2. Have the patient flex and extend their upper extremities against resistance.
3. Have the patient abduct and adduct upper extremities against your resistance.

4. Have the patient flex and extend their forearms against resistance.
5. Have the patient flex and extend their wrists against resistance.
6. Have the patient abduct and adduct their fingers against your resistance.
7. Have the patient adduct their thumbs against your resistance.
8. Passively flex and extend the upper extremities to assess tone.

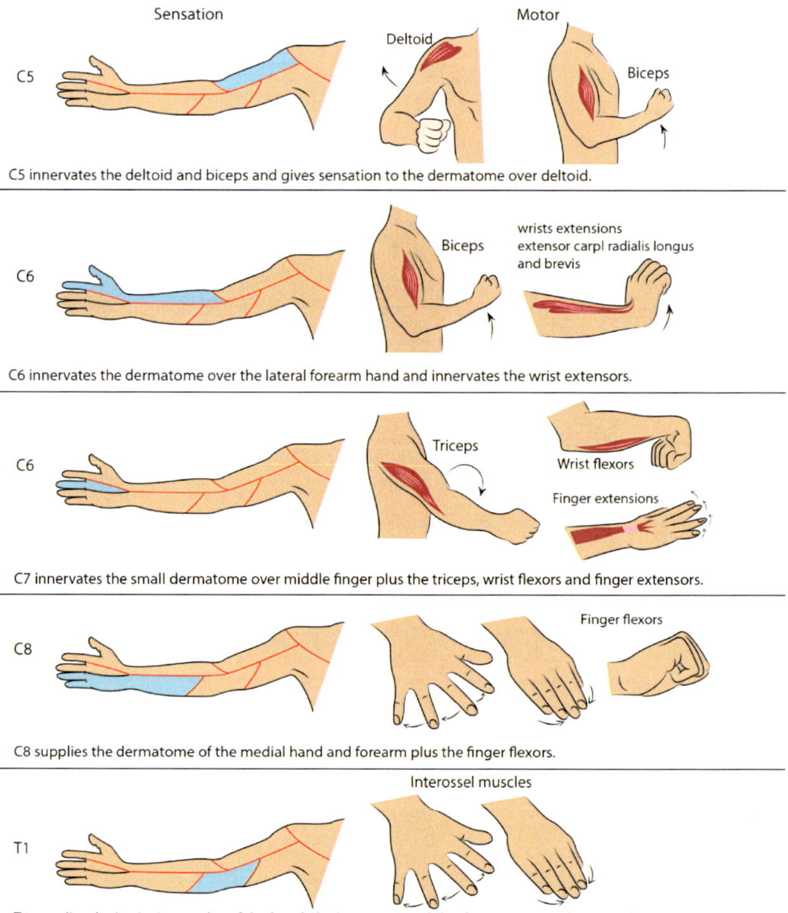

C5 innervates the deltoid and biceps and gives sensation to the dermatome over deltoid.

C6 innervates the dermatome over the lateral forearm hand and innervates the wrist extensors.

C7 innervates the small dermatome over middle finger plus the triceps, wrist flexors and finger extensors.

C8 supplies the dermatome of the medial hand and forearm plus the finger flexors.

T1 supplies the intrinsic muscles of the hand, the interossei, and the dermatome on the medial upper arm.

Level	Motor signs (weakness)
C5	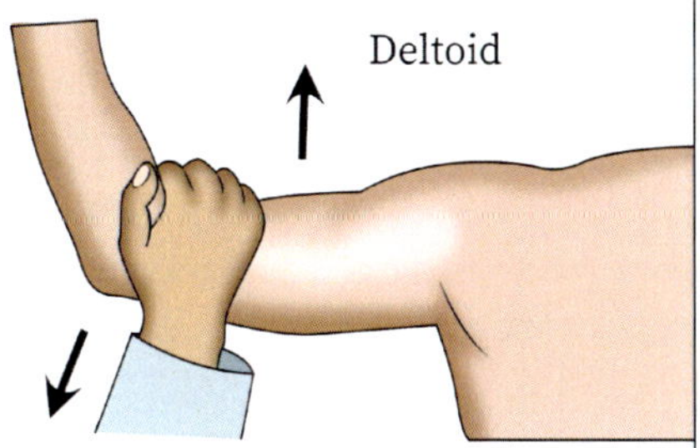
C6	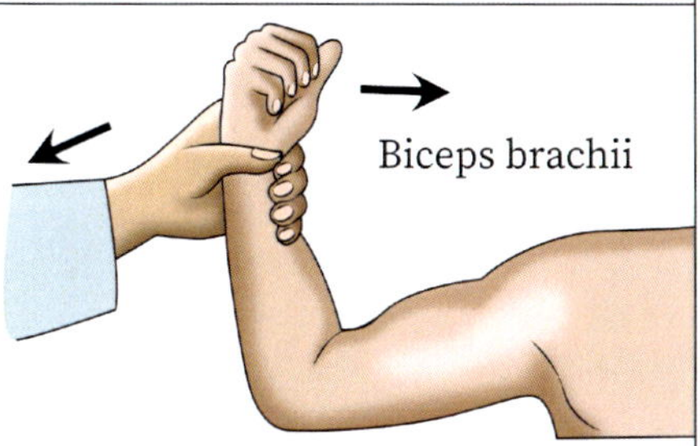
C7	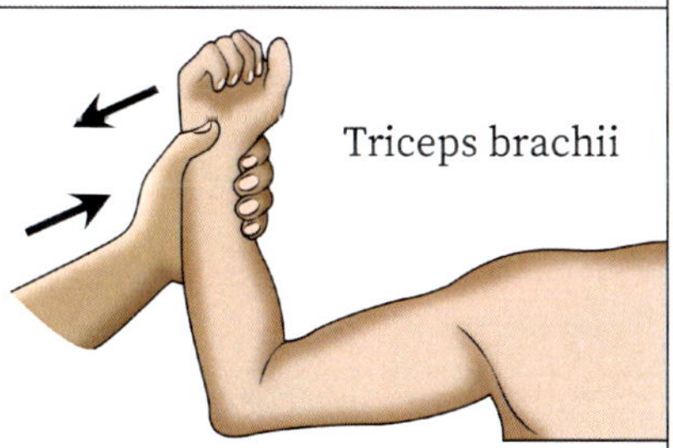
C8	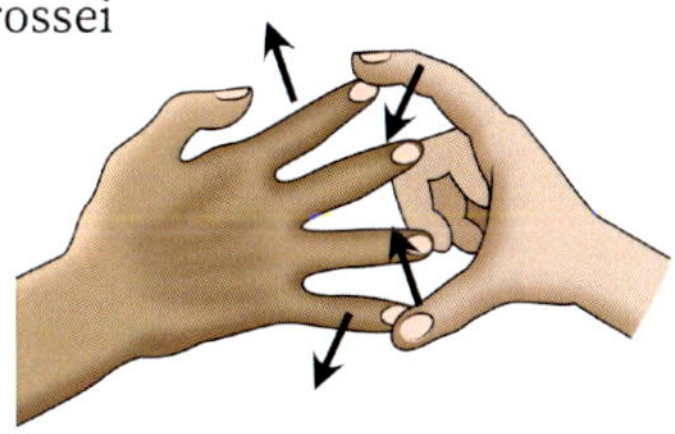

LOWER EXTREMITIES

1. Inspect the lower extremities for symmetry.
2. With the patient lying supine, have them abduct and adduct their hips against your resistance.
3. Have the patient flex and extend their knees against resistance.
4. Have the patient flex and extend their ankles against resistance.
5. Have the patient flex and extend their great toes against resistance.
6. Passively flex and extend the lower extremities to assess tone.

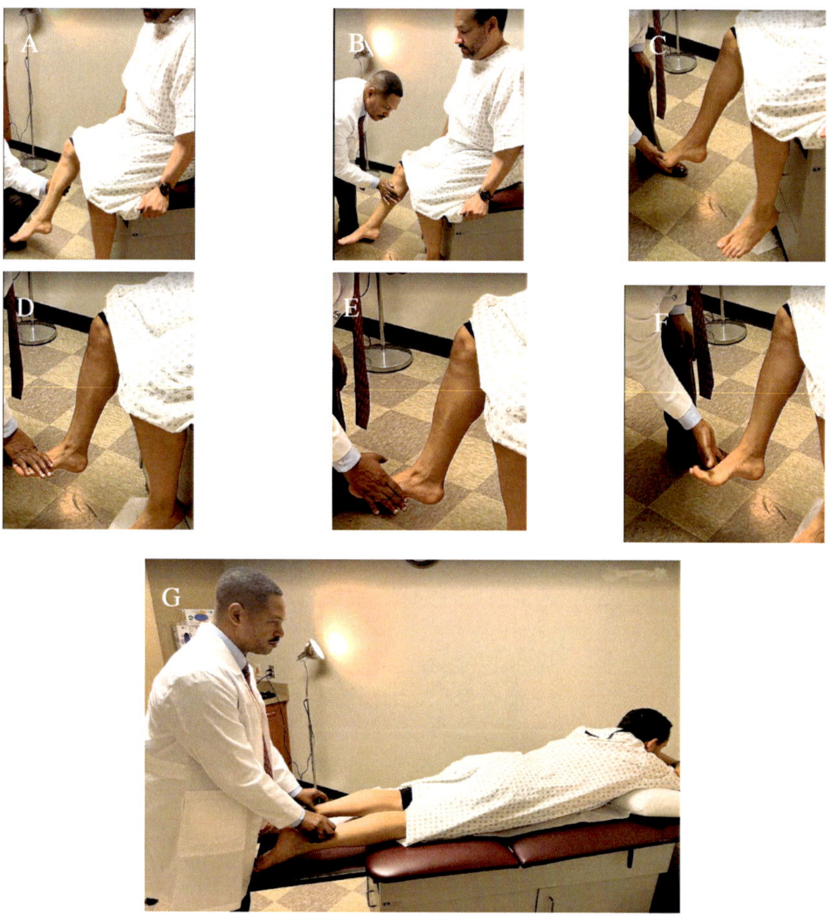

EXAMINATION OF REFLEXES

Two types of reflexes are tested - stretch (deep tendon) and superficial reflexes. It is essential to support patient's joint being tested so that muscles are relaxed.

Hold your reflex hammer between the thumb and index finger and swing from flexion of wrist not the elbow. A gentle tap of hammer pointed at tendon being tested should produce muscle contraction. Reflexes should be symmetrical and equal. Start with the patient sitting.

Tendon Reflexes & Segmental Innervation of the Upper Limb Muscles

- Biceps, brachii tendon reflex
  - C5 & C6
  - Flexion of the elbow joint
  - Tapping on the biceps tendon
- Triceps Tendon Reflex
  - C6-C8
  - Extension of the elbow joint
  - Tapping on the triceps tendon
- Brachioradialis Tendon Reflex
  - C5-C7
  - Supination of the radioulnar joint
  - Tapping the brachioradialis tendon

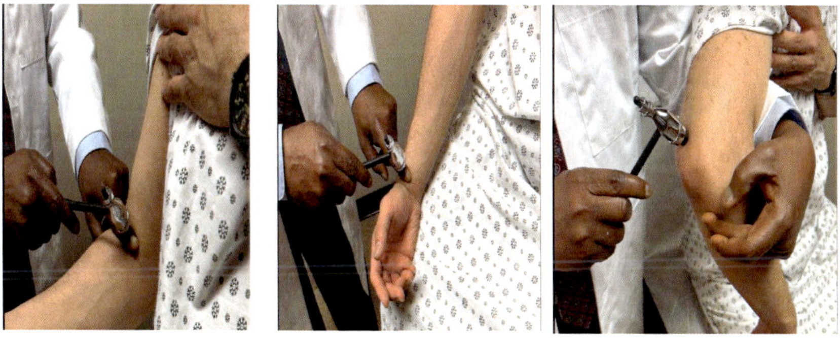

BICEPS

Have the patient relax their arm and pronate the forearm between flexion and extension. Place your thumb over the biceps tendon. Strike your thumb with the hammer.

BRACHIORADIALIS

Have the patient rest their forearm in semiflexion and semipronation on their leg. Strike the styloid process of the radius, about 1-2 inches above the wrist and observe for flexion at the elbow and supination of the forearm.

TRICEPS

Flex the patient's forearm at the elbow and pull the arm toward the chest. Strike the triceps tendon above the insertion of the ulna's olecranon process, about 1-2 inches above the elbow. If a reflex can't be elicited, try to hang the patient's arm over your arm and then strike the triceps tendon.

STRETCH (TENDON TAP) REFLEXES OF LOWER EXTREMITY

PATELLAR

Place you hand on the patient's quadriceps muscle and strike the patellar tendon. You should feel the quadriceps contract and observe the knee extend.

ACHILLES

Place your hand under the patient's foot to dorsiflex their ankle. Strike the Achilles tendon just above its insertion on the posterior aspect of the calcaneus. Observe plantar flexion at the ankle. (The leg needs to be flexed at the hip and knee.)

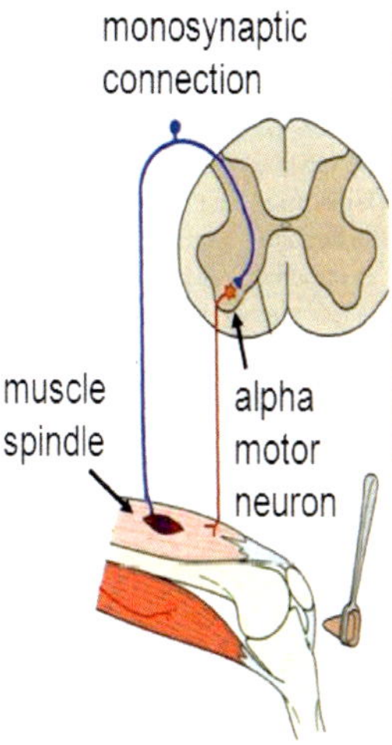

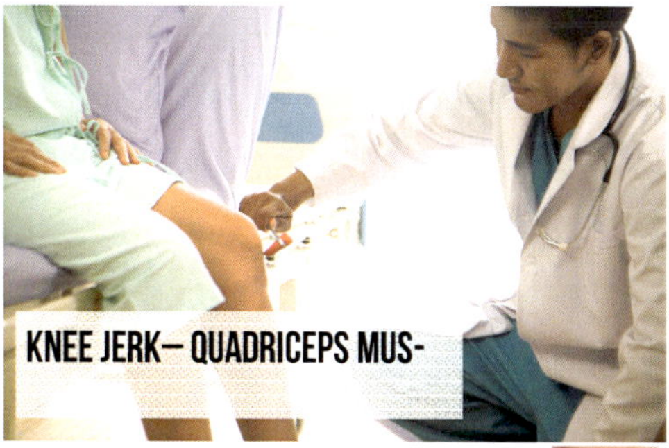

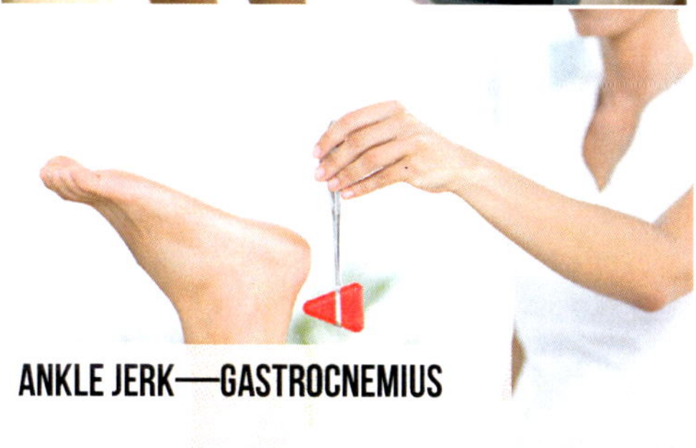

TENDON TAP (STRETCH OR DEEP TENDON) REFLEXES - TEST SPINAL LEVEL

CLINICAL - Patient has numbness of skin overlying little toe. Ankle jerk reflexes reduced. What spinal level affected? S1

BABINSKI

Babinski Reflex

The neurologist Joseph Babinski described the Babinski reflex (plantar reflex) in 1896. The Babinski reflex tests the integrity of the corticospinal tract (CST).

The CST is a descending fiber tract originating from the cerebral cortex through the brainstem and spinal cord. Fibers from the CST synapse with the alpha motor neuron in the spinal cord and help direct motor function. The CST is considered the upper motor neuron (UMN), and the alpha motor neuron is considered the lower motor neuron (LMN). Sixty percent of the CST fibers originate from the primary motor cortex, premotor areas, and supplementary motor areas. Then, about forty percent originates from primary sensory areas, the parietal cortex, and the operculum. Damage anywhere along the CST can result in the presence of a Babinski sign. Stimulation of the lateral plantar aspect of the foot (S1 dermatome) normally leads to plantar flexion of the toes (due to stimulation of the S1 myotome). The response results from nociceptive fibers in the S1 dermatome detecting the stimulation. Nociceptive input travels up the tibial and sciatic nerve to the S1 region of the spine and synapses with anterior horn cells. The motor response that leads to the plantar flexion is mediated through the S1 root and tibial nerve. The toes curl down and inward. Sometimes, there may be no response to stimulation. This is called a neutral response. This response does not rule out pathology.

Babinski sign occurs when stimulation of the lateral plantar aspect of the foot leads to extension (dorsiflexion or upward movement) of the big toe (hallux). Also, there may be fanning of the other toes. This suggests that the sensory input has spread beyond the S1 myotome to L4 and L5. An intact CST prevents such spread. In infants with CST, which is not fully myelinated, the presence of a Babinski sign in the absence of other neurological deficits is considered normal up to 24 months of age. Babinski's may be present when a patient is asleep. The Babinski reflex is done as part of the routine neurological exam and is utilized to determine the integrity of the CST. The presence of a Babinski sign suggests damage to the CST. The only contraindication to performing the Babinski reflex is a lesion (such as an infection) in the affected foot area that precludes the reflex's effective performance. In such situations, other methods can be used.

NEUROLOGICAL ASSESSMENT FINDINGS

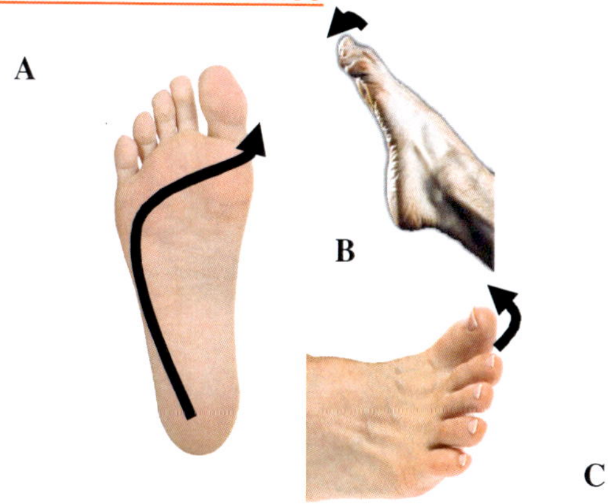

Babinski Response

- A pathological reflex associated with damage to the cortio-spinal tract is the extensor plantar response or the Babinski sign.
- Physiology: one of a group of primitive relexes, including sucking, that are suppressed but reemerge when disorders occur.
- **Note:** The Babinski sign (extensor plantar response) is a normal finding in infants. This response can be found in children from infancy up through two years of age.

NORMAL ADULT RESPONSE—flexion of toes.

Babinski's reflex.

Fig. A. Test maneuver: Using a blunt point, scratch the sole of the foot as shown,

Fig. B, Normal response (absence of Babinski's response) is plantarflexion of the toes.

Fig. C, Abnormal response (presence of Babinski's response) is dorsiflexion of the big toe and often a fanning of the other toes.

EXAMINATION OF SENSORY FUNCTION

LIGHT TOUCH

Ask the patient to close their eyes. Lightly touch patient with a small piece of gauze or cotton. They should tell you when the touch is felt. Compare symmetric points.

PAIN SENSATION

Demonstrate on the patient's hand with, a safety pin or comparable **disposable** sharp object, and say "This is sharp, and this is dull." Ask the patient to close their eyes and respond by saying sharp or dull when a touch is felt. Patient's eyes should be closed.

VIBRATION SENSE

Tap your 128 Hz tuning fork and place it on a bony prominence distally (e.g., distal phalanx of the finger). Instruct the patient to tell you when the vibration is no longer felt.

PROPRIOCEPTION

Hold the distal phalanx of either hand on lateral aspects and move digit up and down explaining to the patient which direction it is being moved. Have the patient close their eyes and move the digits up and down, stopping movement of digit and ask, "Which direction is this, up or down?"

TACTILE LOCALIZATION

Have the patient close their eyes and identify where double touch is felt simultaneously.

TWO-POINT DISCRIMINATION

Gently hold 2 pins 2-3 mm apart and touch patient's fingertip. Ask patient to state the number of pins felt.

STEREOGNOSIS

Ask the patient to close their eyes and identify object placed in hand.

POINT LOCALIZATION

Have patient close eyes. Touch the patient. Ask patient to open eyes and point to area that was touched.

SENSORY FUNCTION-POSTERIOR COLUMN TRACT

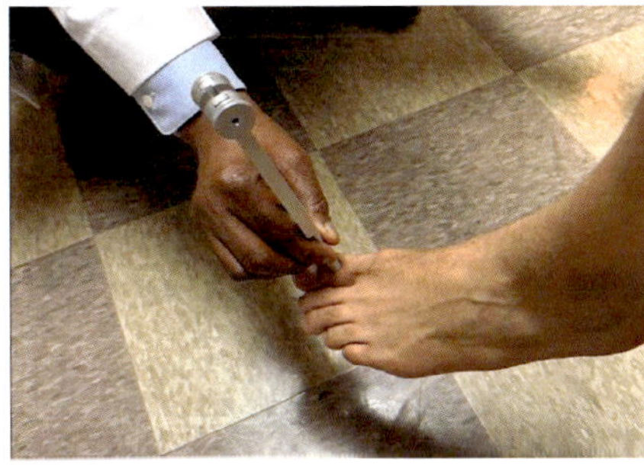

Deep Sensation

Vibration

- Use low pitch tuning fork (128 or 256 Hz)
- Place over bony surface of fingers and great toe

Vibration intact

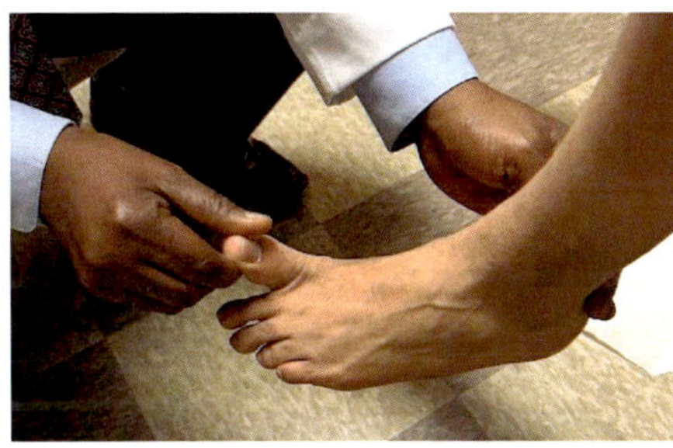

Position (Kinesthesia)

- Move finger or big toe up or down and ask which way it moved

Kinesthesia intact

EXAMINATION OF THE CEREBELLAR FUNCTION

SENSORY FUNCTION SPINOTHALAMIC TRACT

Superficial sensation

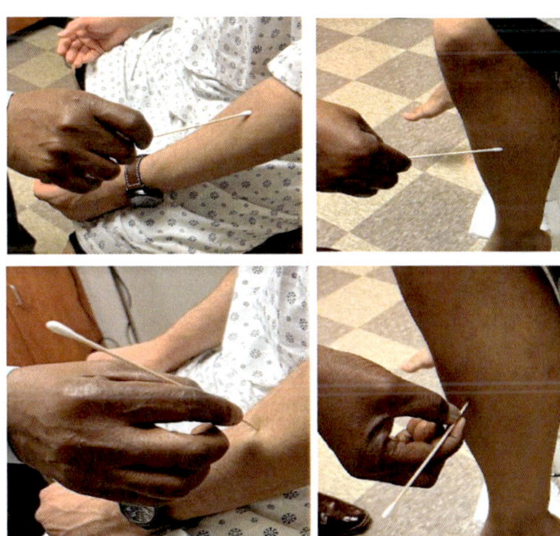

Pain
Assess sharp and dull
Allow at least 2 sec between

Temperature
Text only when pain sensation abnormal

Light (crude) touch
Apply wisp of cotton to arms, forearms, hands, chest, thigh, an legs

Sharp and dull and light touch intact

Palm Rotation

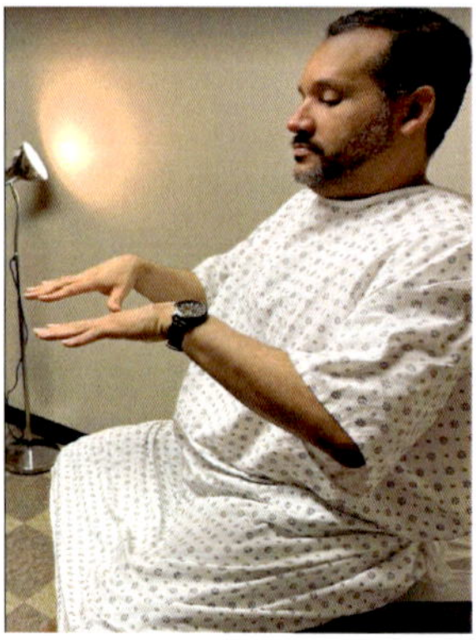

Heel to Shin Test

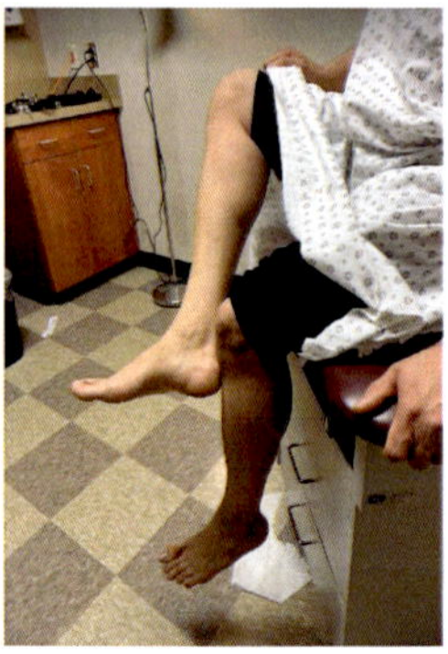

Dysdiadochokinesia Test

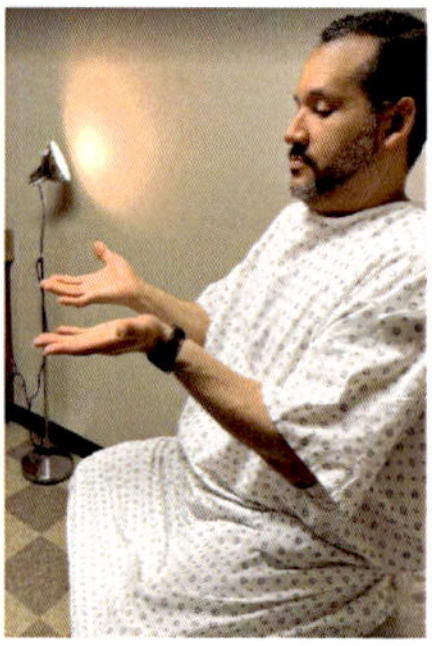

Finger to Nose Test

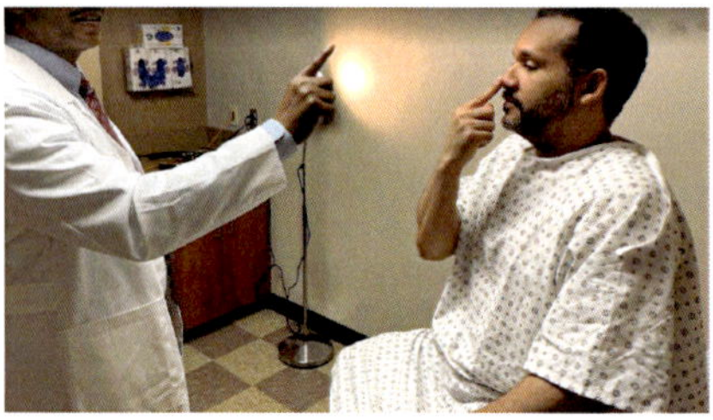

Clinician's Index Finger

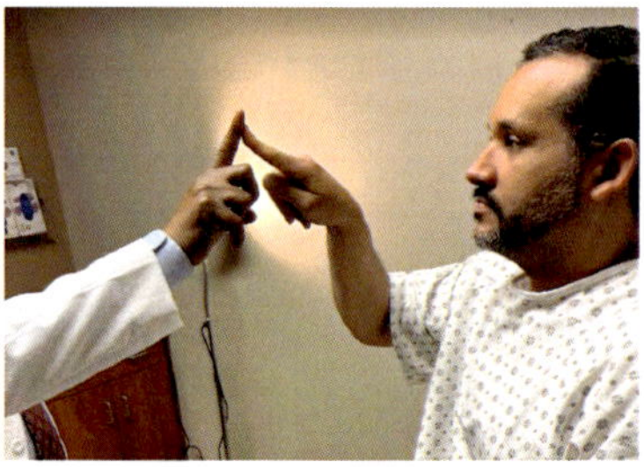

1. Finger to nose test: Ask the patient to stretch out their arms and close their eyes. Then, have them touch the tip of their nose with each index finger, alternating hands and increasing speed
2. Heel to knee test: Ask the patient to place their heel on the opposite knee and run it down the shin to the ankle in supine position (Not over clothing).
3. Rapid alternating movements: Ask the patient to pronate and supinate their hands against their thighs, increasing in speed.
4. Romberg's test: Have the patient stand in front of you and put their feet and toes together. Ask them to extend their arms with their palms facing up and close their eyes. You should stand next to the patient in case they start to fall.
5. Gait: Ask the patient to walk across the room. Also walk in front of the patient with your arms spread apart while observing the patient's gait. This is done to prevent fall of the patient.

EXAMINATION OF THE ABDOMEN

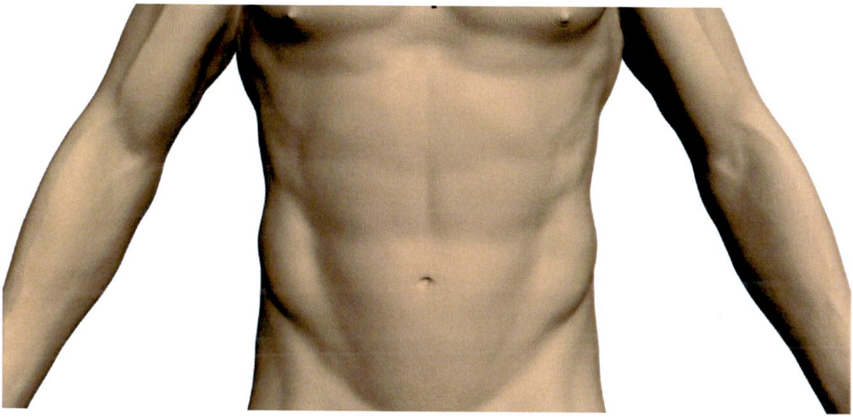

SCAN TO SEE ABDOMEN EXAM

BRIEF INTRODUCTION

The major components of the abdominal exam include inspection, auscultation, percussion, and palpation. When looking, listening, feeling and percussing, imagine what organs live in the area that you are examining. The abdomen is roughly divided into four quadrants: right upper, right lower, left upper and left lower. By thinking in anatomic terms, you will remind yourself of what resides in a particular quadrant and therefore what might be identifiable during both normal and pathologic states.

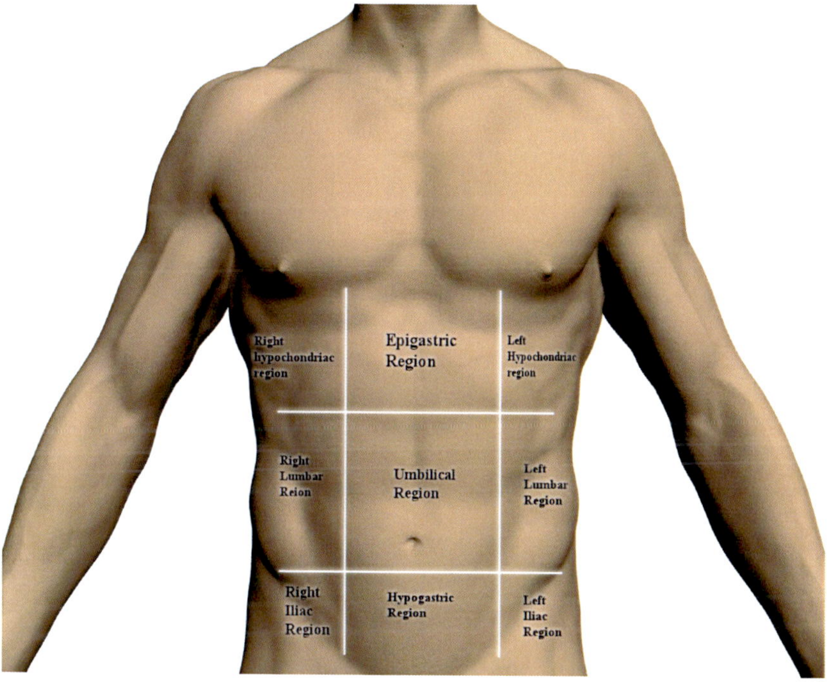

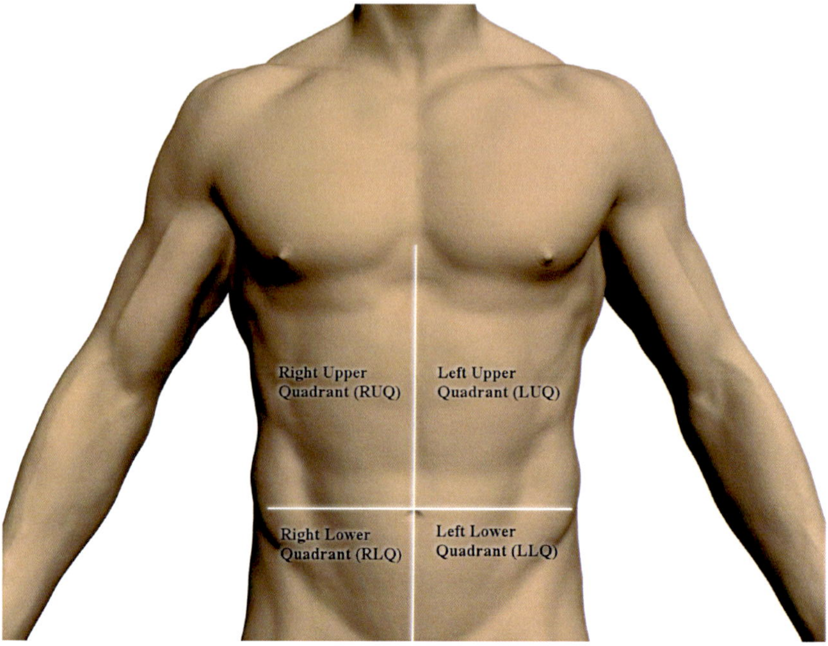

GOALS

Student should be able to physically examine the abdomen using:

1. Inspection
2. Auscultation
3. Percussion
4. Palpation

PERFORMANCE OBJECTIVES

1. Inspect the abdomen region
2. Identify the abdominal topographic anatomy landmarks
3. Identify the organs found in each abdominal quadrant (epigastrium, periumbilical, and hypogastric areas)
4. Auscultation the abdomen demonstrating the appropriate technique
5. Percussion of the abdomen demonstrating the appropriate technique
6. Percuss the liver (estimate the size of the liver)

7. Perform light and deep palpation of the abdomen demonstrating the appropriate technique

INSPECTION

1. Stand on the right side of the bed with the patient in the supine position, legs flat, and arms at the side.
2. Ensure patient is comfortable, pillow under head, chest drape, and table extension is pulled out.
3. Drape chest, expose abdomen fully, and assess patient comfort level from the xyphi-sternum to the pubic symphysis.
4. Observe the contour of the abdomen while standing on the right side of the patient.
5. Stand near the foot of the bed and observe the symmetry of abdomen contour (have the patient breathe deeply).
6. Ask patient to lift head and shoulders off bed (check for abdominal hernia) or cough strongly.
7. Observe aortic pulsation.
8. Inspect skin for: color, scars, lesions, striae, distention, and hair distribution.

AUSCULTATION

1. Assure that your stethoscope is warm.
2. Place stethoscope on the skin with just enough pressure to assure good contact.
3. Start in the right lower quad and listen to bowel sounds.
4. Proceed to listen in all four quads.
5. Assess and document the frequency and pitch of the sounds.
6. If bowel sounds are absent you must listen for a full 5 minutes, over the abdomen, before concluding and charting that bowel sounds are not present. (If you do not hear bowel sounds during the skills assessment you will need to state that you would normally listen for 5 minutes to conclude that bowel sounds are truly absent.)

7. Use the bell, pressing gently over the abdomen, starting in the epigastric region at the aorta, renal, iliac, and femoral arteries.

ABDOMINAL EXAMINATION AUSCULTATION

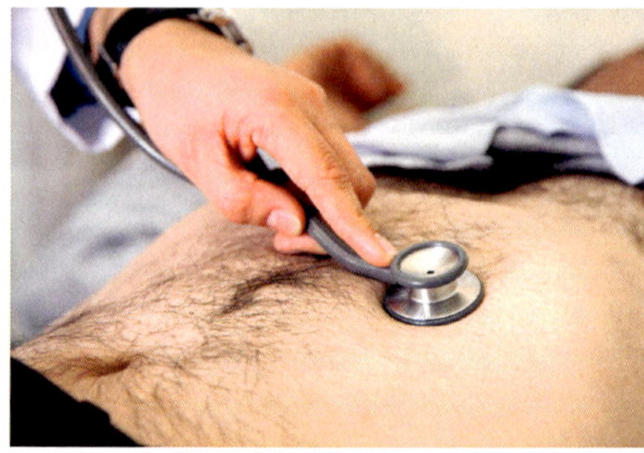

Place the diaphragm of the stethoscope to the right of the umbilicus

Bowel sounds (borborygmi) are caused by peristaltic movements

Occur every 5-10 sec.

Absence of b.s.: paralytic ileus or peritonitis

Bruits over aorta and renal a. could be a sign of an aneurysm and stenosis

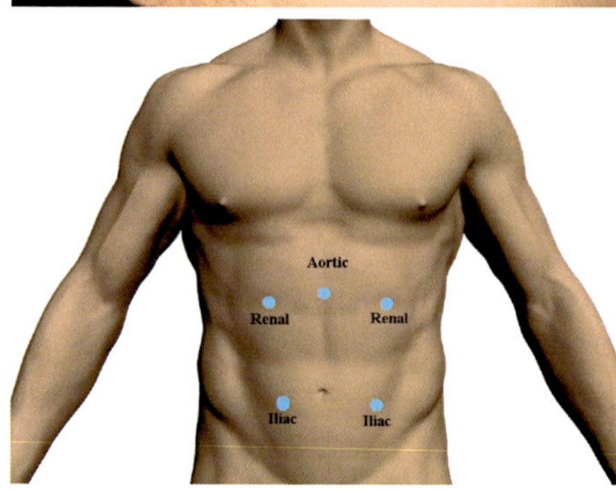

ABDOMINAL PERCUSSION

1. Percuss lightly in each quadrant (Tympany usually predominates).
2. Percuss in all 9 areas of the abdomen. Percussion techniques may vary. A circular, continuous, horizontal or vertical technique may be used.
3. Percuss over areas of unexpected bulging.

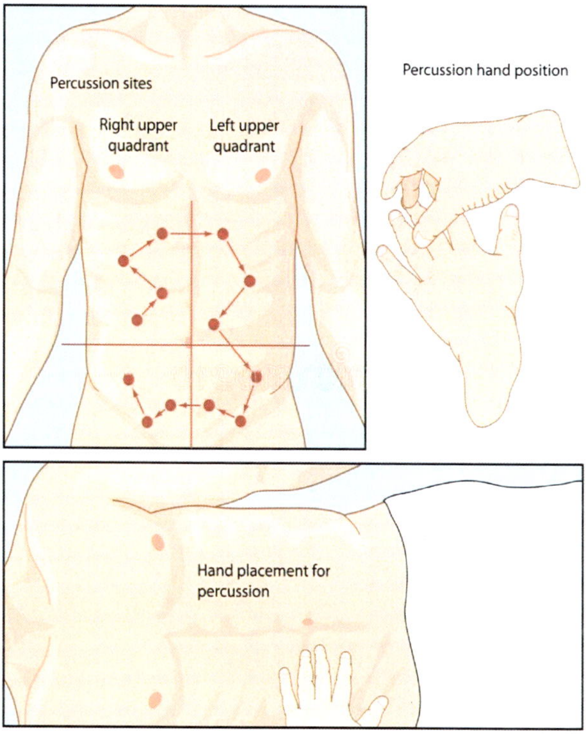

SHIFTING DULLNESS

1. Percuss from the umbilical area downward toward the flank in several directions horizon to the mid line.
2. To map the lateral borders, note the change from tympany to dullness.
3. Roll patient onto one side; percuss and identify the border again.

LIVER PERCUSSION

1. Percuss in the right midclavicular line starting in the mid chest. Percuss from area of resonance to area of dullness in 1 -inch steps. **Mark this point.**
2. Locate lower border by percussing upward beginning at the level of the umbilicus. Percuss from tympany to dullness in 1 inch step beginning at the level of the umbilicus. **Mark this point.**
3. Measure the distance between the 2 points in the midclavicular line (6 to 12 cm is normal).
4. If the liver seems enlarged percuss from midsternal and anterior axillary lines.

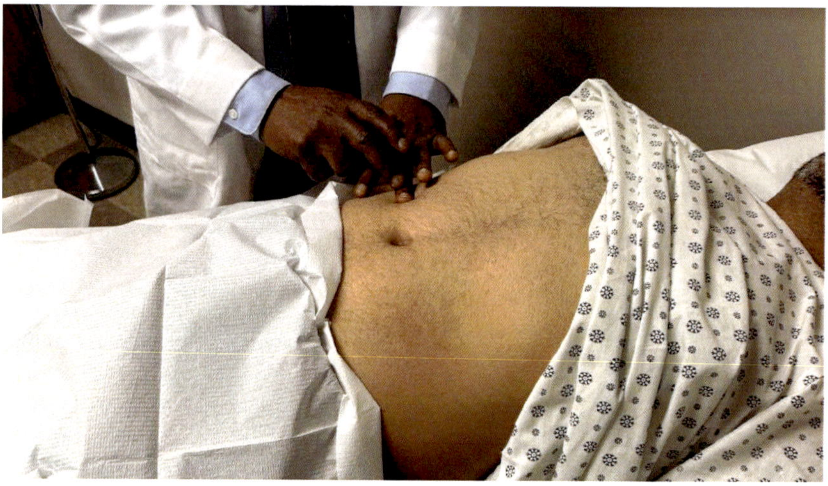

PALPATION OF THE ABDOMEN

1. Warm your hands.
2. To aid in relaxation of the abdomen, place a pillow beneath the knees.
3. Palpate any area of tenderness last.

LIGHT PALPATION

1. Palpate with first four fingers close together. Depress the skin about 1 cm making a gentle rotary motion.
2. Slide fingers and skin together, lifting the fingers and move clockwise to the next location around the abdomen.
3. Hand and arm are parallel to the abdominal skin.
4. Observe patient's face for any signs of discomfort.
5. If stomach wall is tense, have patient flex knees.

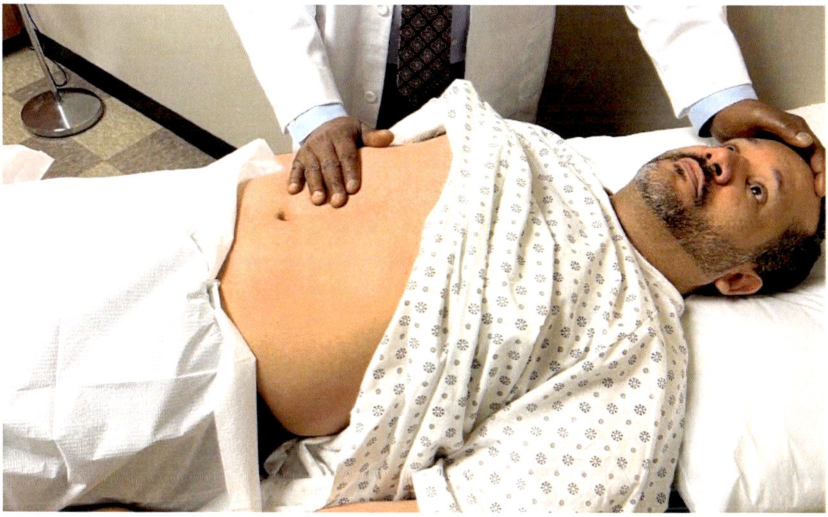

DEEP PALPATION

1. Palpate with a two-handed technique.
2. Place one hand down on the abdomen and place the other hand over it.
3. Use the top hand to press down while feeling the structures with the other hand.
4. Palpate through each quadrant.
5. Mass — Describe and document depth, size, shape, location, consistency, and tenderness. If you cannot tell if it is in the wall or not, have the patient tense their abdomen.
6. (Masses in the abdominal wall will remain palpable).

LIVER (BIMANUAL) PALPATION

1. Stand on the patient's right side.
2. Place left hand posteriorly between patient's right 12th rib and iliac crest.
3. Place right hand near the umbilicus, lateral to the rectus abdominus muscle.
4. Always begin low in case the liver is enlarged.
5. Aim fingers vertically or obliquely to patient's upper left.
6. Lift left hand up slightly and press slightly in with right hand.
7. Have patient breathe deeply and feel for the liver edge as it descends. If you do not feel the edge of the liver, bring your right hand up 1 inch and try again. (The liver edge is usually not palpable.)
8. If you feel the edge of the liver, check for tenderness.
9. **Check for Murphy's sign**. A catch in the respiration is a positive finding, strongly suggestive of Acute Cholecystitis.

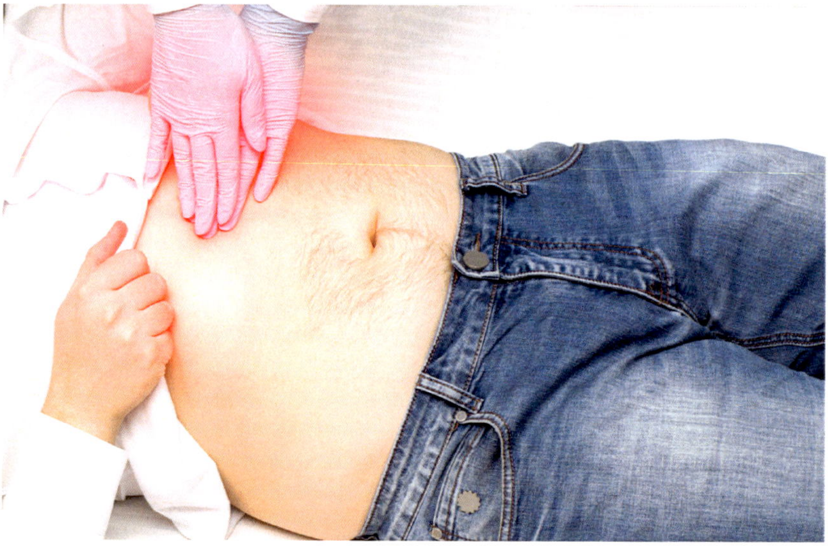

ALTERNATE (HOOKING) MANEUVER

1. Stand above the patient, facing toward feet.
2. Place both hands, side by side, below the right costal margin.
3. Ask patient to inhale deeply and curl fingertips inward and upward under the patient's rib cage.

ALTERNATE METHOD

Liver Palpation

- Stand by the patient's chest
- "Hook" your fingers just below the costal margin and press firmly.

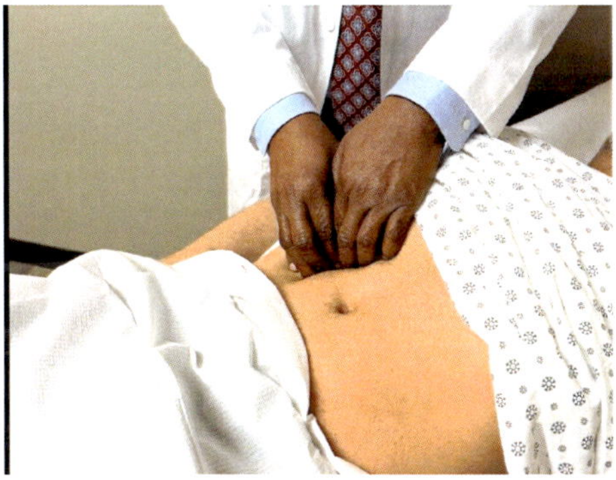

SPLEEN

1. Stand to the patient's right side.
2. Reach with your left hand over and under the patient's left posterior inferior costal margin
3. Place your right hand near the umbilicus.
4. With fingers aimed upward, toward the patient's spleen, lift up with the left hand to displace the spleen anteriorly.
5. Ask the patient to breathe deeply while palpating for the spleen.
6. If palpable, describe and document the edge in cm below the left costal margin.
7. If enlarged, roll the patient to right side with knees and hips slightly flexed and try palpation again.

RIGHT KIDNEY

1. Place left hand under flank.
2. Place right hand below the right costal margin with the fingertips positioned toward the midline.
3. Ask patient to inhale deeply.
4. With left hand lift upward while right hand depresses deeply. The lower pole may be felt as a smooth rounded mass as it descends during inspiration.

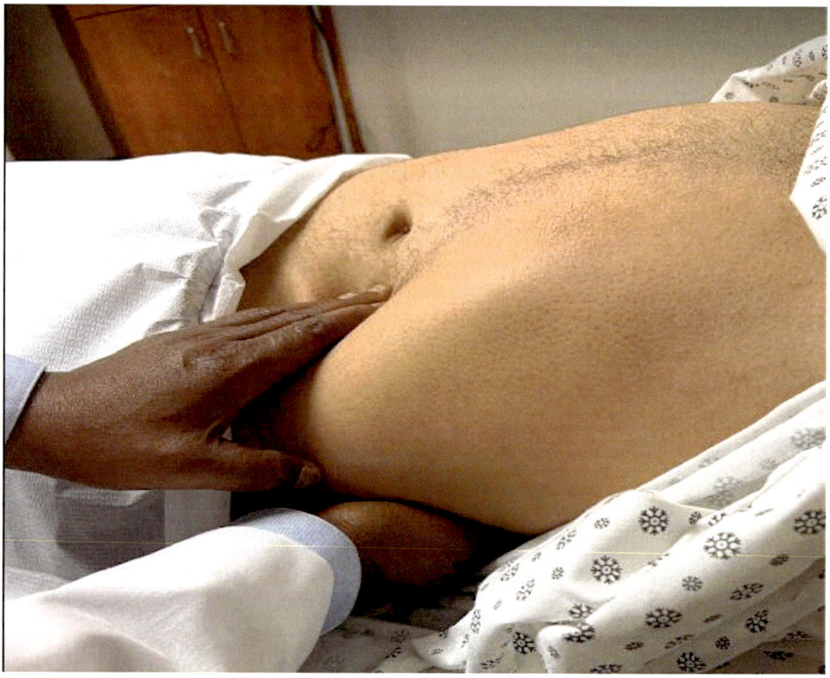

LEFT KIDNEY

1. Remain on the patient's right side.
2. Reach with left hand over and under patient's left posterior inferior costal margin.
3. Place right hand near the umbilicus aiming fingertips more toward the left flank.
4. Ask patient to inhale deeply.

5. With left hand lift upward while right hand depresses deeply. The lower pole may be felt as a smooth rounded mass as it descends during inspiration.

AORTA

1. Press the fingertips of the right hand deeply but gently into the epigastric area slightly left of the midline.
2. Gauge the width of the pulsation.
3. Encircling with thumb and fingers, press gently.
4. Describe and document the aorta pulsation (aorta is 2.5 to 4 cm wide).
5. Note: Alternate technique for obese individuals; using both hands press fingertips deeply in on both sides of the aortic pulsation

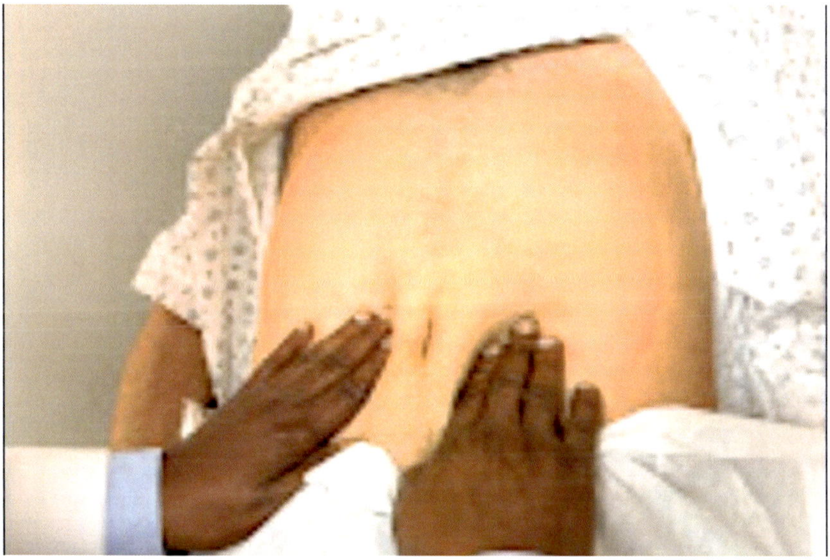

REBOUND TENDERNESS

1. Hold hand 90 degrees to the abdomen and press the fingertips firmly, but slowly, into the abdomen near the area of suspicion or pain.
2. **Release quickly.** (If there is **rebound tenderness**, there will be pain upon release of your hand.)
3. Have the patient point to the pain.

ROVSING'S SIGN

1. Press in the left lower quadrant. Sudden release will cause pain in the right lower quadrant (Indicative of appendicitis).

MCBURNEY'S POINT

1. Tenderness in the right lower quadrant is a sign of localized peritoneal irritation. From the right anterior superior Iliac spine locate one-third medial and from the umbilicus locate two-third lateral, that point is called McBurney's, indicative of appendicitis.

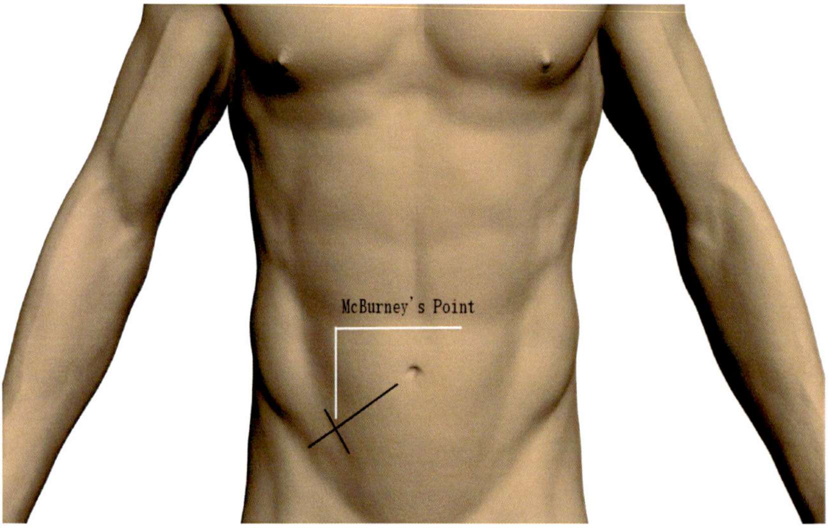

OBTURATOR SIGN

1. Flex the right knee and hip 90 degrees (upon the chest).
2. Grasp the ankle and rotate the hip internally and externally.
3. Intrapelvic inflammation will cause lower-quadrant pain on the affected side. This discomfort indicates a positive test result.

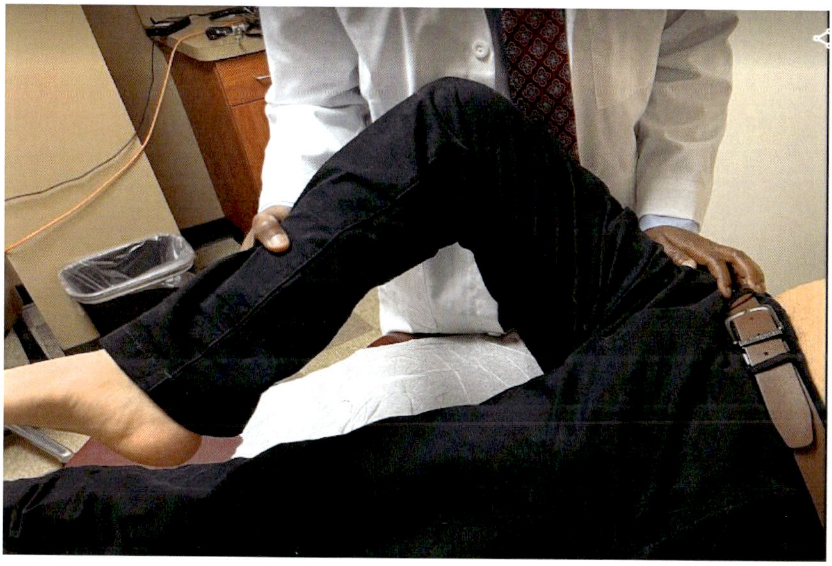

PSOAS SIGN

1. Ask patient to raise a straightened right leg against resistance.
2. Alternatively, ask patient to lie on left side and the examiner gently hyperextends straightened leg to stretch the psoas major muscle.

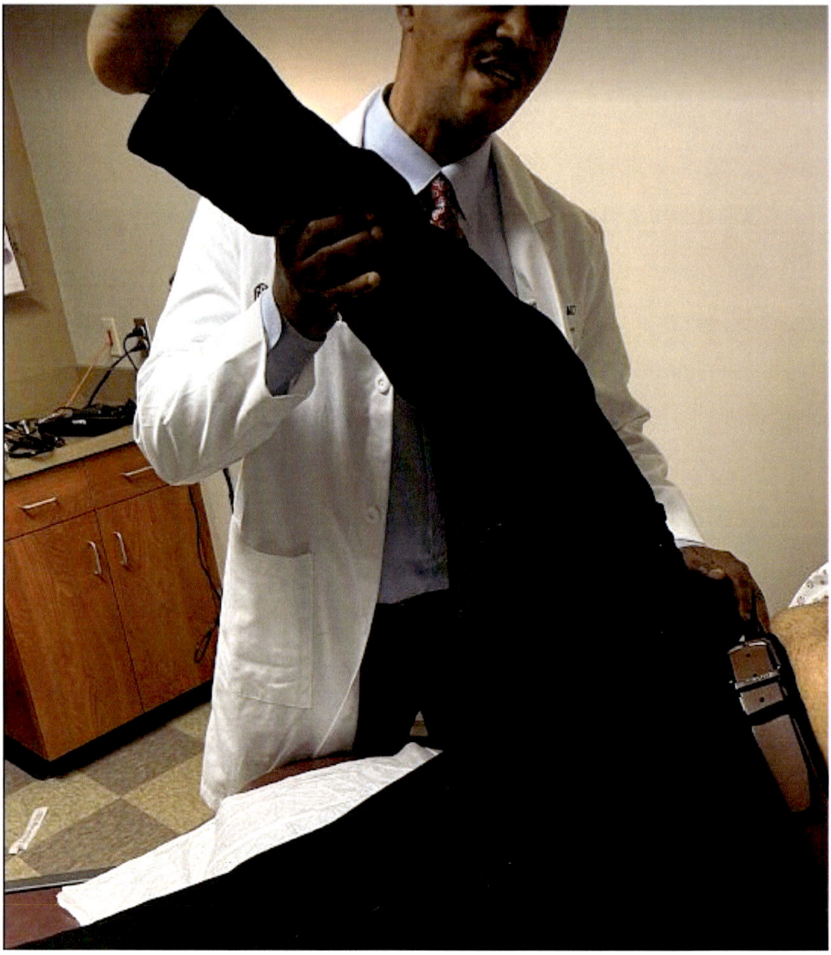

RENAL TENDERNESS

1. Place patient in sitting position.
2. Place fingers over the costovertebral angle and lightly palpate. If there is no pain, place left palm over one costovertebral angle.
3. Percuss lightly.
4. Percuss firmly with right fist (check each side).

Note: Rectal Exam concludes the abdominal exam, but it is not done in standardized patient.

MUSCULOSKELETAL SYSTEM EXAM

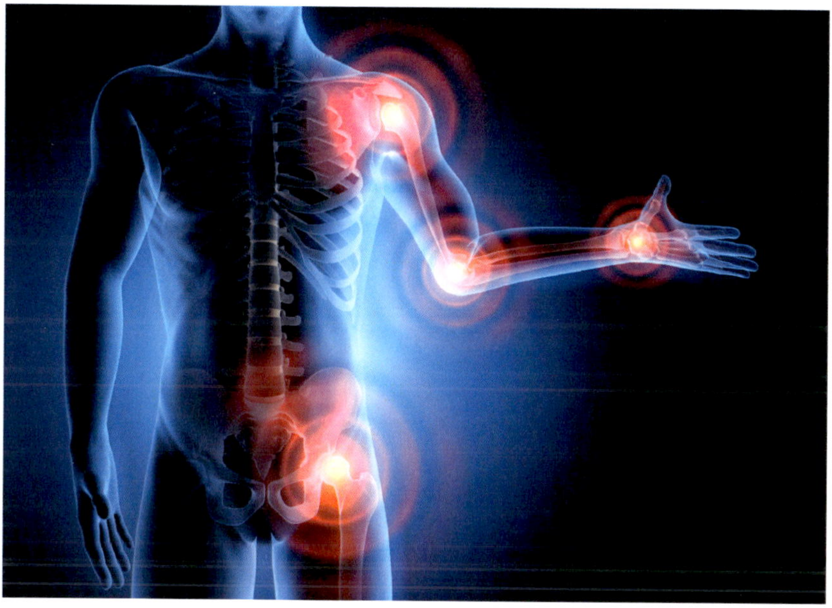

SCAN TO SEE MOTOR FUNCTION TEST

BRIEF INTRODUCTION

The function of the Musculoskeletal system (Musculo—muscles; Skeletal– bone, tendons and cartilage) is to conduct movement and coordination of the body. Most hospital visits to a primary physician office involves the complain of the musculoskeletal.

The examination of the musculoskeletal system involves examination of: a. spinc, b. Temporomandibular joint, c. arm, d. hand, e. hip, leg and foot. Inspecting all those areas (a, b, c, d, e,), palpation of all those areas (a, b, c, d, e,),, assessing of the movement of all those areas (a, b, c, d, e,),. Also, in some of the areas like arm, and the leg examining for sensation, deep tendon reflexes and peripheral pulses may be necessary to complete the musculoskeletal system.

GOALS

Upon completion of these exercises the learner should be able to:

1. Comprehend the procedures for examining the musculoskeletal system.
2. Physically examine the musculoskeletal system by palpating common evaluation techniques.
3. Recognize musculoskeletal abnormalities.
4. Be familiar with motor function to cord segment.

PERFORMANCE OBJECTIVES

1. Demonstrate proper techniques for inspection, palpation and manipulations of major muscle groups and joints
2. Perform different tests and techniques used to asses functions of joints and regions of musculoskeletal system
3. Perform a basic musculoskeletal; examination correlating anatomical concepts

EXAMINATION OF TEMPORAL MANDIBULAR JOINT (TMJ)

1. Palpate the temporomandibular joint by placing the index fingers bilaterally, anterior to the tragus of the ear. Have patient clinch teeth to palpate the masseter muscle.
2. Instruct patient to open and close mouth slowly. The range of motion should feel smooth and gliding. There should be no tenderness, pain or audible clicking.

TMJ EXAMINATION

Palpation of the TMJ

A. Lateral aspect of the joint with the mouth closed.
B. Lateral aspect of the joint during opening and closing.
C. With the patient's mouth fully open, the clinician moves a finger behind-the condyle to palpate the posterior aspect of the joint.

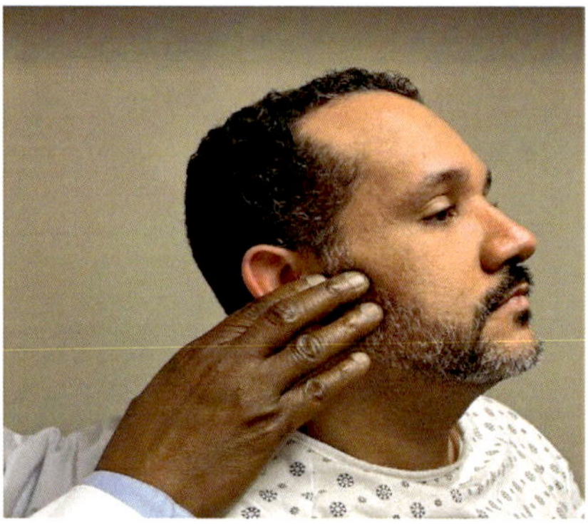

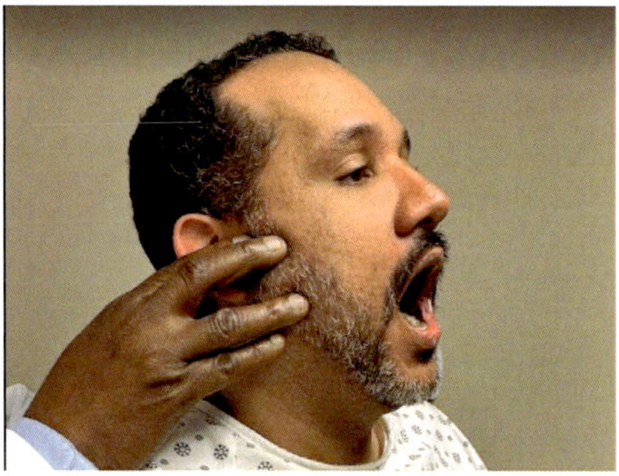

CERVICAL SPINE EXAMINATION (NOT OVER CLOTHES)

1. Inspect patient's cervical spine noting any bony abnormalities.
2. Palpate the spinous process noting any abnormal protrusions, insertions, or tenderness.
3. Palpate the paraspinal musculature.
4. Perform active range of motion (AROM) of the cervical spine (cervical flexion, extension, rotation, and side flexion).
5. Perform cervical spine motion against resistance.

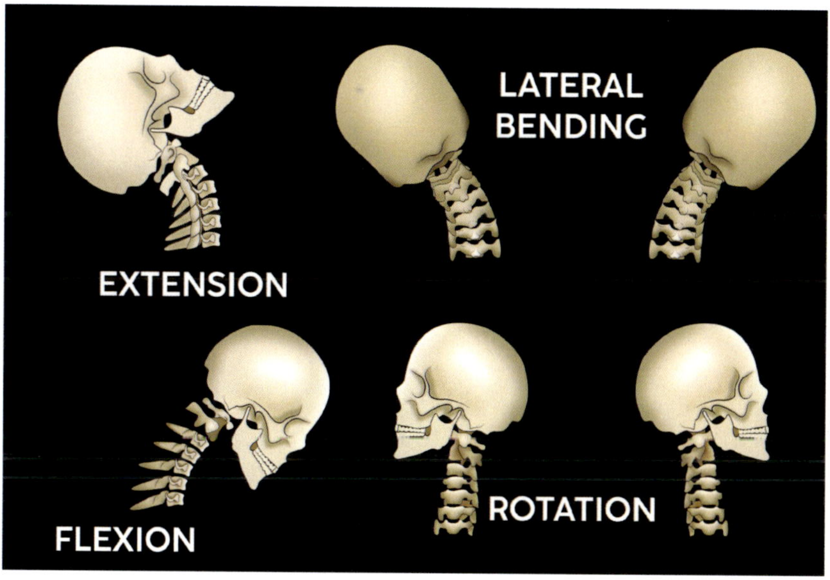

SHOULDER EXAMINATION

1. Inspect the shoulders bilaterally noting any wasting of musculature, bony defects (e.g. winging of the scapula), or swelling of soft tissue.
2. Palpate the shoulder complex consisting of the acromioclavicular, sternoclavicular, and costo-sternal joints. (Crepitus, pain, tenderness,)

3. Perform active range of motion (AROM) of the shoulder complex.
4. Instruct the patient to abduct the arms fully and place palms together above the head. Arms should come close to touching patient's ears in the vertical position. Ask patient to place their hands on their back between the scapulae. Hands should normally reach the level of the inferior angle of the scapulae. This maneuver also tests internal rotation of the humerus and the range of motion at the elbow.

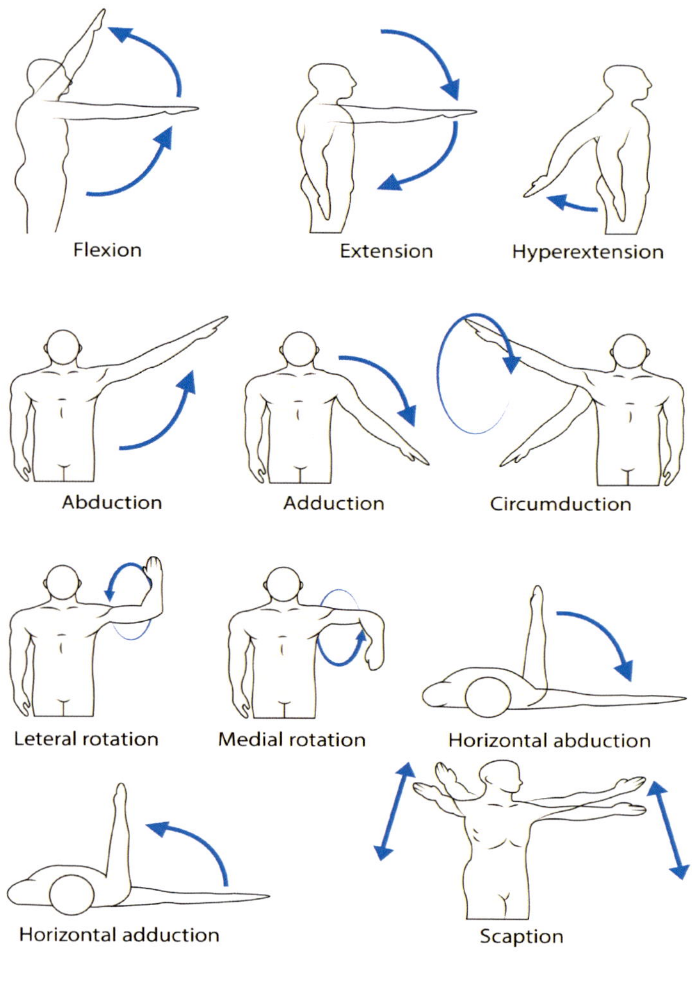

ELBOW EXAMINATION

1. Inspect elbow for deformities, (e.g., dislocation) and swelling.
2. Palpate the medial and lateral epicondyles as well as the olecranon of the ulna.
3. Ask patient to rotate forearm checking for supination/ pronation.
4. Ask patient to flex and extend arm at the elbow against resistance while stabilizing the elbow.
5. Palpation of the radial and brachial pulses.
6. Performing DTR for triceps, biceps and brachioradialis muscles.

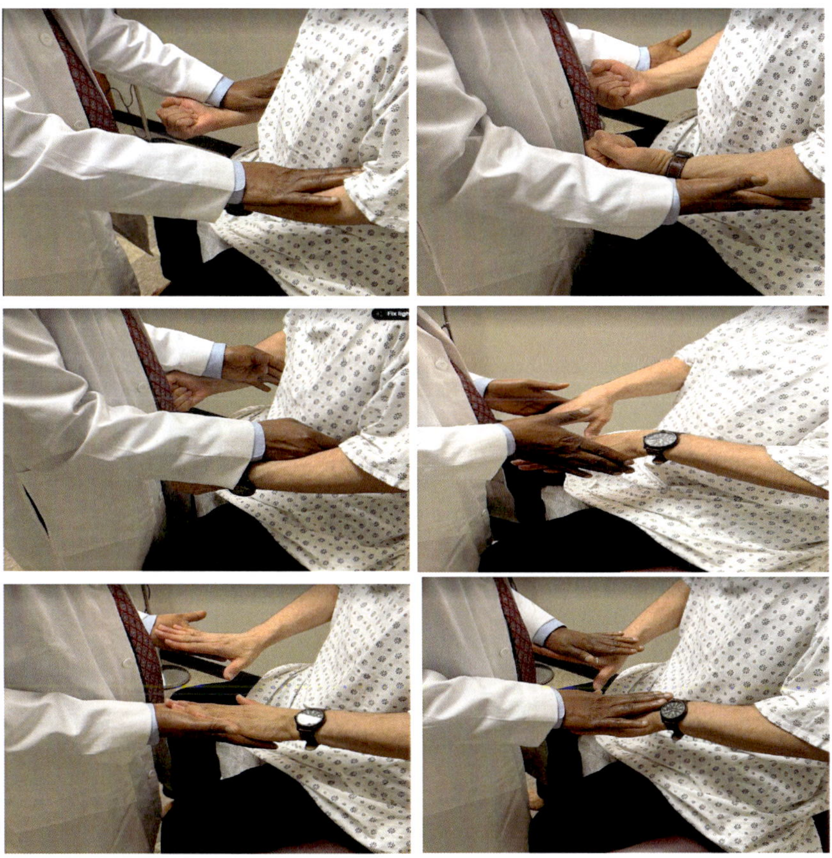

HAND EXAMINATION

1. Inspect and examine the fingernails, pads, thenar/ hypothenar, Interosseous and joints (DIP-distal interphalangeal joint, PIP-proximal interphalangeal joint and MCP – metacarpophalangeal joint) musculature.
2. Check capillary refill time. Perform this by pressing the nail bed and noting how long it takes for the nail bed to become pink again. Normal capillary refill is less than 3 seconds.
3. Check sensory deficits in the radial, median, and ulnar dermatomal distribution. Stroke various regions of patient's hand with your index finger asking patient if there is a difference in sensation. Ideal locations to test for sensation are: the hypothenar region to evaluate the ulnar nerve; the thenar region and distally to evaluate the median nerve; the anatomical "snuff box" located dorsal surface to evaluate the radial nerve.
4. Palpate the metacarpophalangeal (MCP), Proximal (PIP) and Distal Interphalangeal (DIP) joints between your thumb and index finger as well as patient's wrist joints, noting any tenderness, swelling, or redness (ulnar deviation is found in severe Rheumatoid Arthritis).
5. Examine the function of the hand. Evaluate extension, flexion, adduction and abduction of the wrist (radial nerve).
6. Thumb opposition ask patient to touch the thumb to each finger individual testing the median nerve.
7. Test the intrinsic of the hand (ulnar). Instruct patient to spread fingers (abduction), attempt to compress the fingers together against resistance (adduction).
8. Test for grip strength instructing patient to grasp examiner's fingers and squeeze gently.

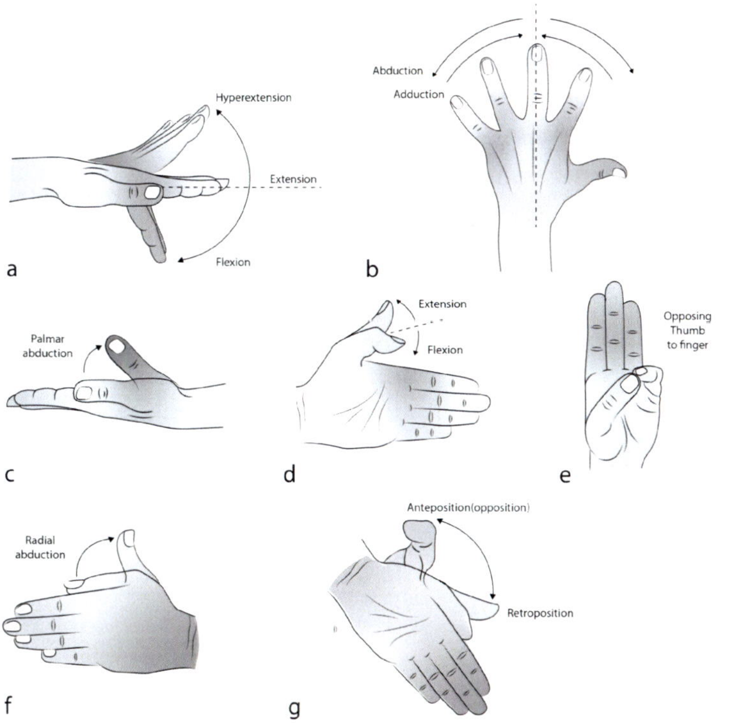

EXAMINATION OF THORACOLUMBAR SPINE

1. Inspection of the spine noting posture and looking for abnormal curvatures or deformities (e.g., scoliosis, kyphosis, and lordosis). Remember you should inspect the spine - anteriorly, posteriorly and laterally.
2. Deeply palpate the thoracolumbar spine and paravertebral muscles for tenderness - noting any bony and soft tissue abnormalities.
3. Test AROM (Active, Range, of Motion) of the spine standing behind patient and stabilizing hips. (Flexion, side flexion, and rotation (circumduction)).
4. Ask patient to lie supine on the exam table.

5. Check AROM for the hip - flexion, extension, abduction and adduction and against the examiner resistance. See figure 5 below for different hip movements.

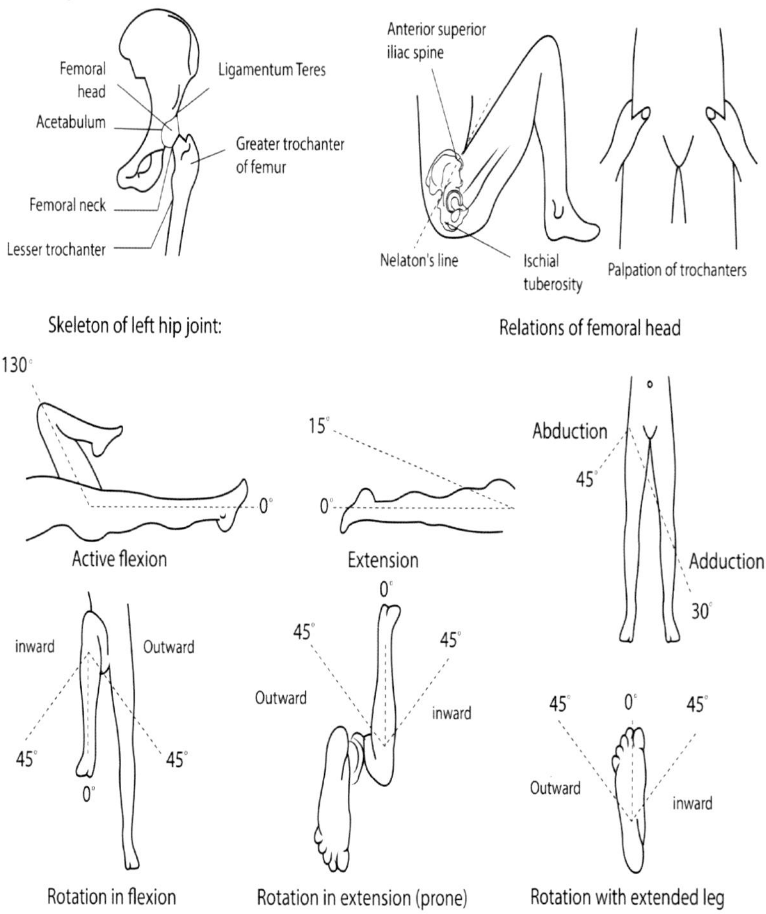

Motion of the Hip Joint

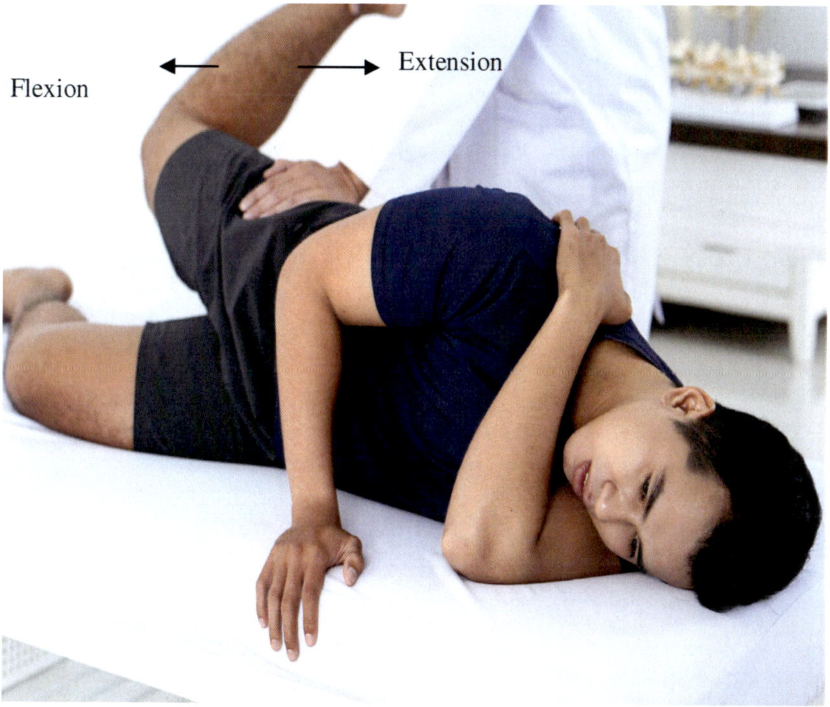
Flexion
Extension

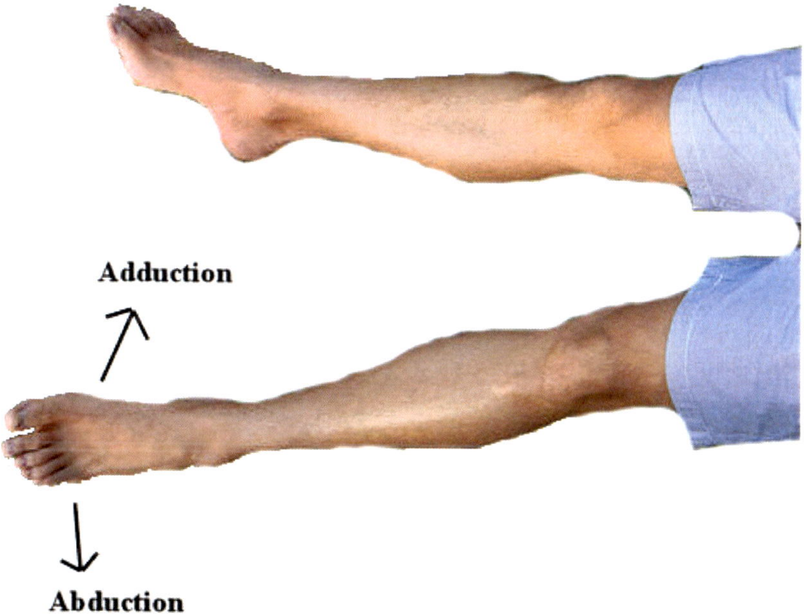
Adduction
Abduction

STRAIGHT LEG TEST

The straight leg raise is a test that can be performed during a physical examination, with the leg being lifted actively by the patient or passively by the examiner. If the straight leg raise is done actively by the patient, it is a test of functional leg strength, particularly the rectus femoris element of the quadriceps (checking both hip flexion and knee extension strength simultaneously). If carried out passively (also called Lasègue test or Lazarević's sign), it is used to determine whether a patient with low back has an underlying nerve root sensitivity, often located at L5 (5th lumbar spinal nerve).

1. Begin with the patient lying down on their back on an examination table or exam floor.
2. The examiner lifts the patient's leg while the knee is straight.
3. A variation is to lift the leg while the patient is sitting. However, this reduces the sensitivity of the test.
4. In order to make this test more specific, the ankle can be dorsiflexed, and the spine flexed. This increases the stretching of the nerve root and dura.
5. If the patient experiences sciatic pain, and more specifically pain radiating down the leg (radiculopathy), when the straight leg is at an angle of between 30 and 70 degrees, then the test is positive, and a herniated disk is a possible cause of the pain. A negative test suggests a likely different cause for back pain.

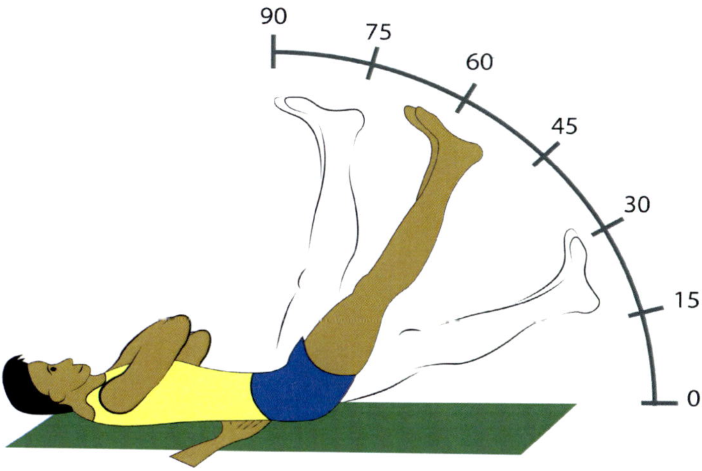

EXAMINATION OF THE KNEE

The **knee examination**, is performed as part of a physical examination or when a patient presents with knee pain or a history that suggests a pathology of the knee joint.
The exam includes several parts:

1. position/lighting/draping
2. inspection
3. palpation
4. motion

The latter three steps are often remembered with the saying **look, feel, move.**

Inspection

1. Make sure that both knees are fully exposed. The standardized patient should be in either a gown or shorts.
2. Inspect for edema, erythema, venous stasis, or vessel abnormalities. These abnormalities can be more pronounced while the patient is standing.
3. When standing, inspect for any evidence of bowing (varus) or knock-kneed (valgus) deformity.
4. Inspect for any asymmetry or scars.

5. Inspect for any atrophy of the quadriceps, hamstring, or calf muscle groups.
6. Ask the patient to walk and inspect for any gait abnormality.
7. Inspect the external anatomy -patella, patella tendon, medial and lateral joint lines, tibial tuberosity, femur and tibia.

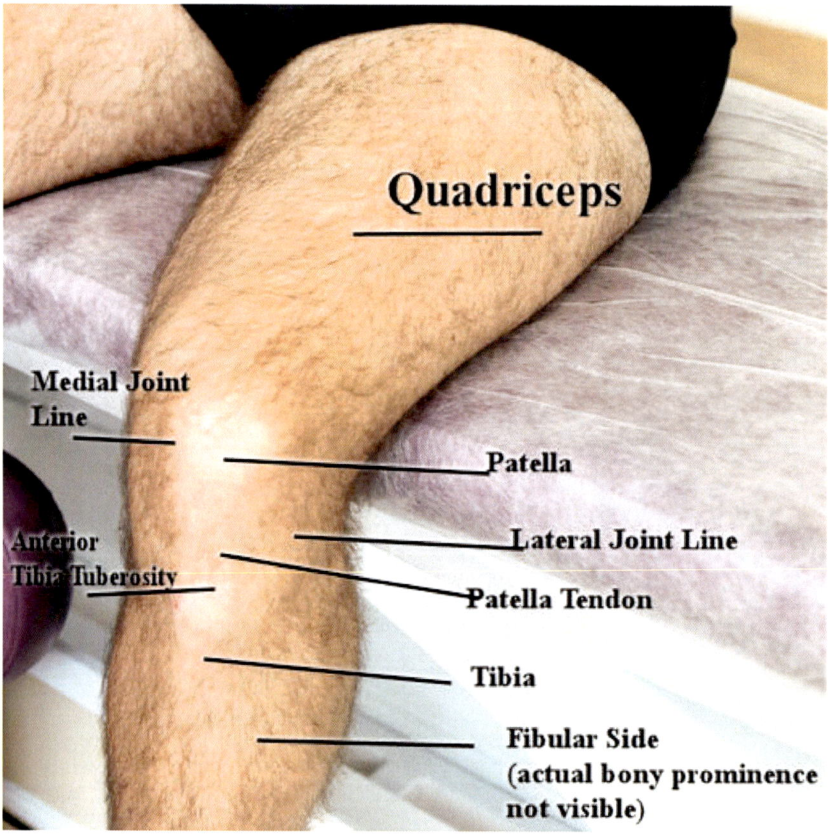

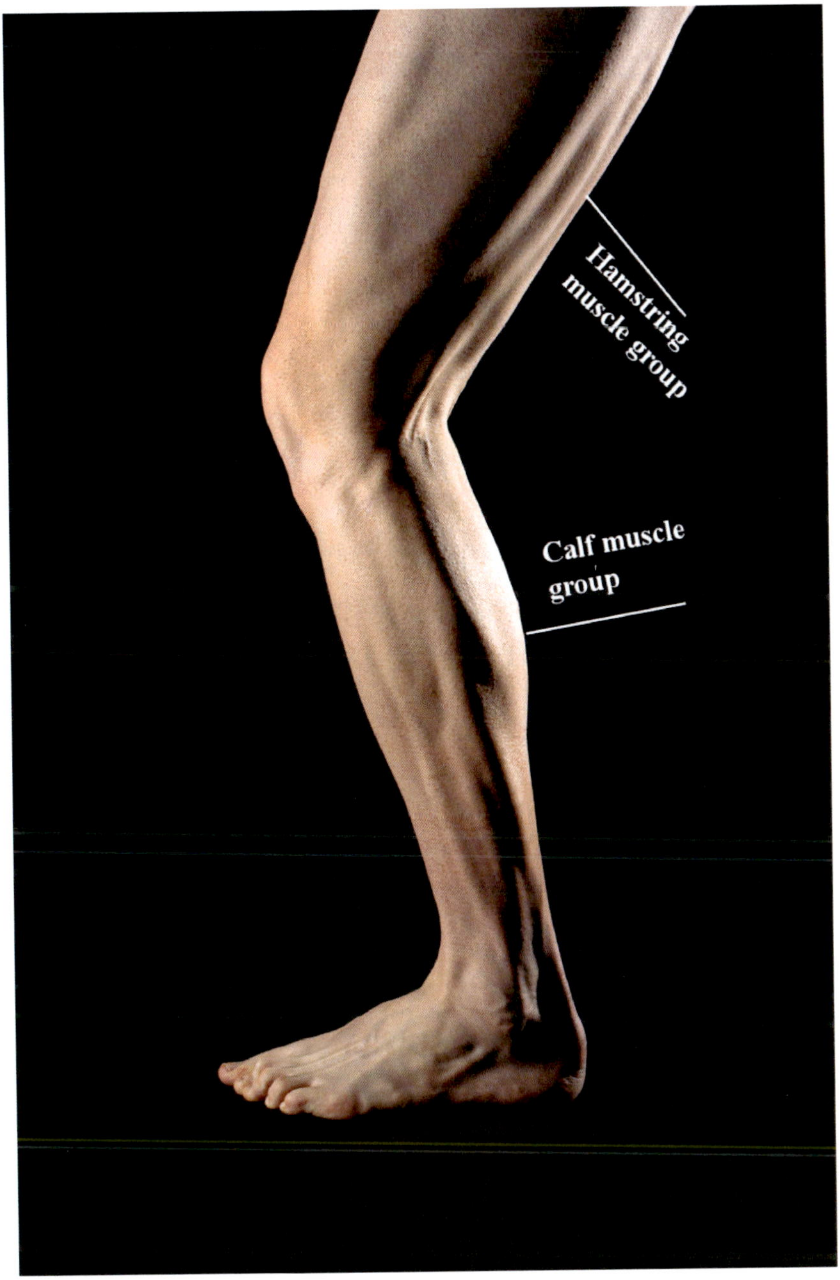
Hamstring muscle group
Calf muscle group

PALPATION OF THE KNEE

1. Start by examining the unaffected side.
2. Palpate the entire joint line of the knee noting any tenderness. Collateral ligaments can be appreciated by pressing thumbs lateral to the patellar tendon beneath the femoral condyles.
3. Ask the patient to bend the knee, gauging whether they can fully extend and flex. This is referred to as their active range of motion. Full extension is 0 degrees, full flexion ~ 140.
4. Place one hand on the patella. Note any warmth, which if present, would suggest inflammation.
5. Grasp the ankle or calf with your other hand and gently flex the knee. Note the extent to which you can flex and extend the knee, referred to as its passive range of motion.
6. Using the hand on the patella, feel for crepitus. This is a crackling/grinding sensation that occurs with movement.
7. Palpate the popliteal fossa. Place thumbs on the patella and the remaining fingers of both hands in the popliteal space behind the knee. Position leg in a mild degree of flexion with the foot resting on the table. Palpate throughout the popliteal fossa noting any fullness or fluctuance (e.g., Baker's cyst).

MOTION

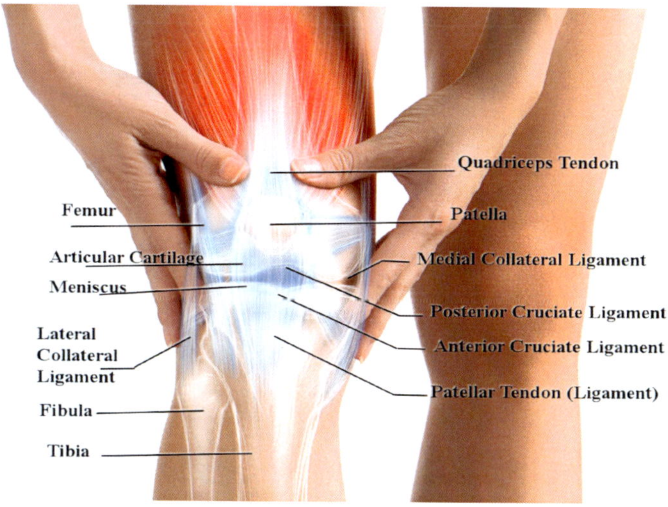

ASSESSMENT OF EFFUSION

1. The absence of normal grooves around patella may indicates a patellar intra-articular effusion.
2. Patellar tap test is used to test for patella effusion - squeeze the fluid between the patella and the femur by pressing at the medial patella using a non-dominant hand. Then, using the dominant hand to press on the patella vertically. If the patella is ballotable, then patellar intra-articular effusion is present.

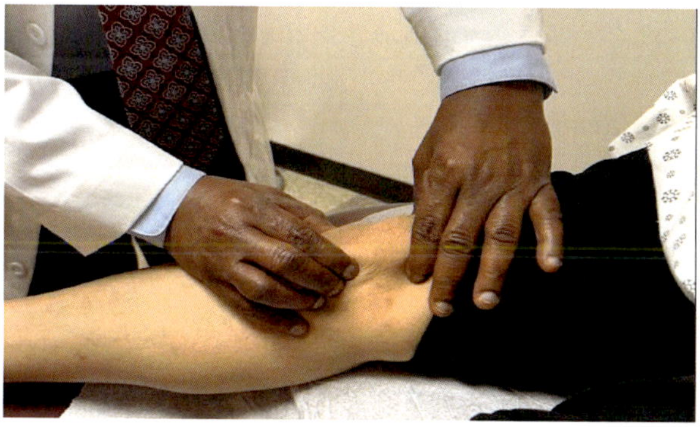

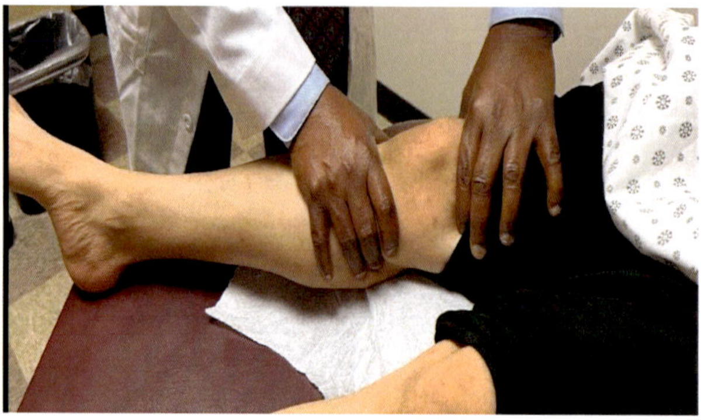

ASSESSMENT OF COLLATERAL LIGAMENTS OF THE KNEE

1. The **valgus stress test** or **medial stress test** is a test for damage to the medial collateral ligament of the knee. It involves placing the leg into extension, with one hand placed as a pivot on the knee. With the other hand placed upon the foot applying an abducting force, an attempt is then made to force the leg at the knee into valgus. If the knee is seen to open up on the medial side, this is indicative of medial collateral ligament damage and may also indicate capsular or cruciate ligament laxity.

2. **Varus Test**: The patient's leg should be relaxed for this test. The examiner should passively bend the affected leg to about 30 degrees of flexion. While palpating the lateral joint line, the examiner should apply a varus force to the patient's knee. A positive test occurs when pain or excessive gapping occurs (**some gapping is normal at 30 degrees**).

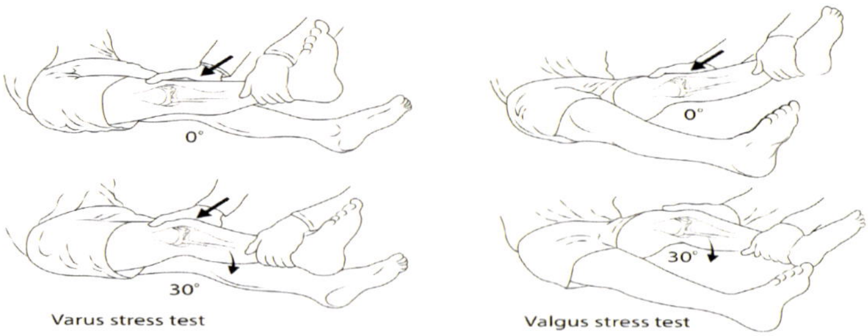

ASSESSMENT OF ANTERIOR CRUCIATE LIGAMENT

The anterior drawer test and Lachman test can be used to access the integrity of the anterior cruciate ligament.

1. The **drawer test** is used in the initial clinical assessment of suspected rupture of the cruciate ligaments in the knee. The patient should be supine with the hips flexed to 45 degrees, the knees flexed to 90 degrees and the feet flat on table. The examiner positions himself by sitting on the examination table in front of the involved knee and grasping the tibia just below the joint line of the knee. The thumbs are placed along the joint line on either side of the patellar tendon. The tibia is then drawn forward anteriorly. An increased amount of anterior tibial translation compared with the opposite limb or lack of a firm endpoint may indicate either a sprain of the anteromedial bundle or complete tear of the ACL If the tibia pulls forward or backward more than normal, the test is considered positive. Excessive displacement of the tibia anteriorly suggests that the anterior cruciate ligament is injured.

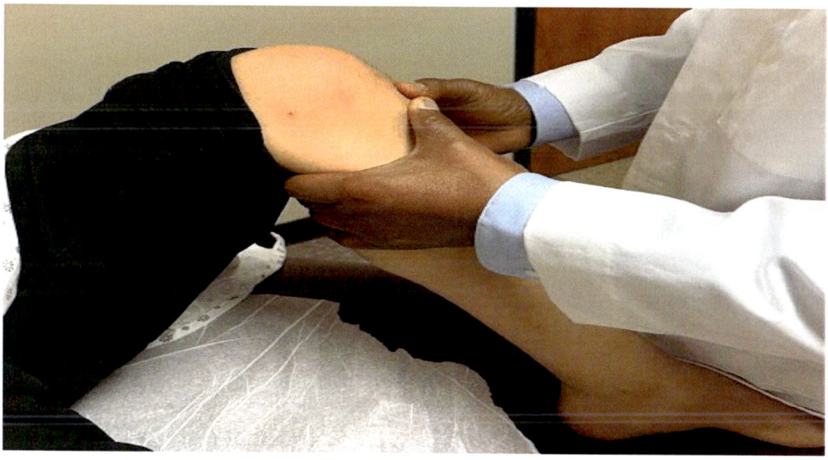

2. The Lachman test is recognized as reliable, sensitive, and usually superior to the anterior drawer test. The knee is flexed at 15 degrees with the patient supine. The examiner should place one hand behind the tibia and the other grasping the patient's thigh. It is important that the examiner's thumb be on the tibial tuberosity. The tibia is pulled forward to assess the amount of anterior motion of the tibia in comparison to the femur. An intact ACL should prevent forward translational movement ("firm endpoint") while an ACL-deficient knee will demonstrate increased forward translation without a decisive endpoint - a soft or mushy endpoint is indicative of a positive test.

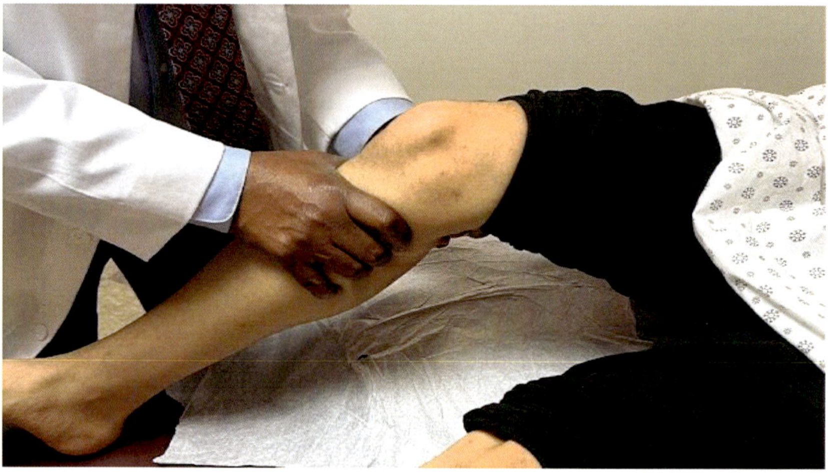

ASSESSMENT OF POSTERIOR CRUCIATE LIGAMENT

1. Posterior drawer test can determine the integrity of the posterior cruciate ligament. Like anterior drawer test, the knee should be flexed 90 degrees and the tibia is pushed backwards. If the tibia can be pushed posteriorly, then the posterior drawer test is positive.

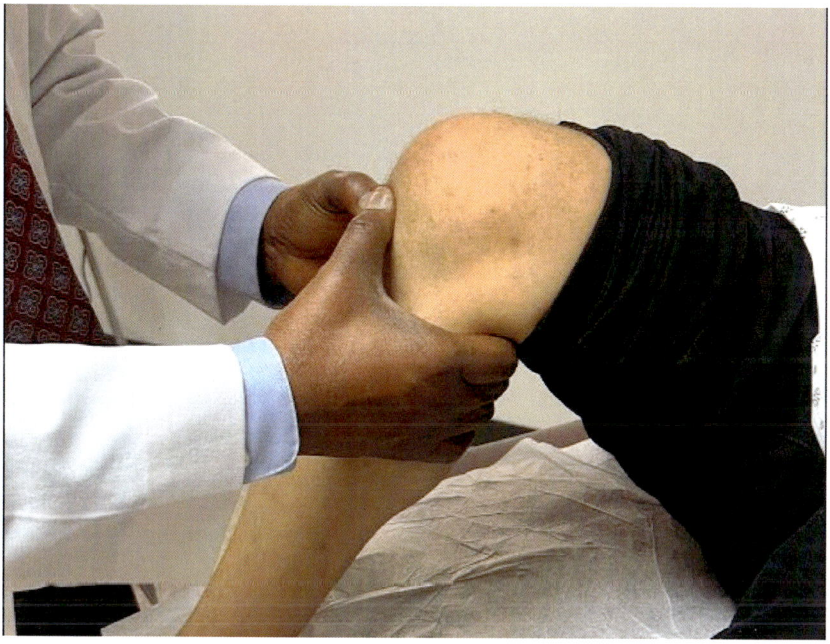

ASSESSMENT OF MENISCUS

Those with meniscal injuries may report symptoms such as clicking, catching, or locking of knees. Apart from joint line tenderness, use the **McMurray test to** assess meniscal tear.

1. Place the patient's tested leg in maximal hip and knee flexion. While palpating the joint line, apply a valgus force to the knee, while simultaneously externally rotating and extending the knee completely. Place the tested leg back in maximal hip and knee flexion. While palpating the joint line, apply a varus force to the knee, while simultaneously inter-

nally rotating and extending the knee completely. A positive test occurs when pain or clicking/thudding is produced.

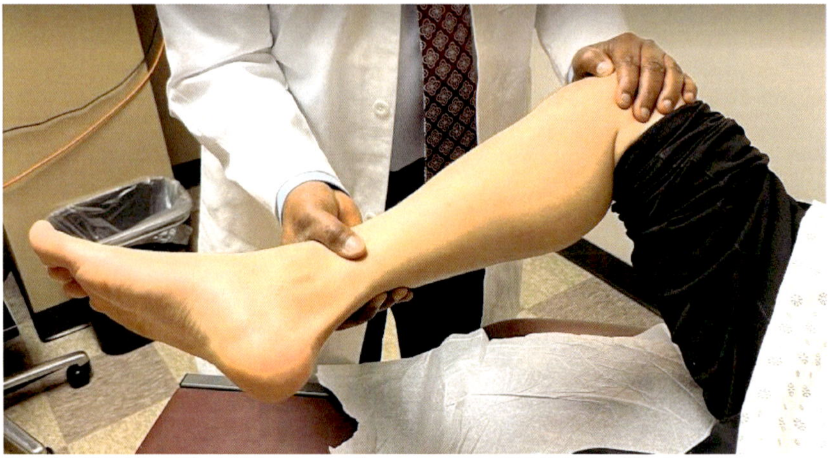

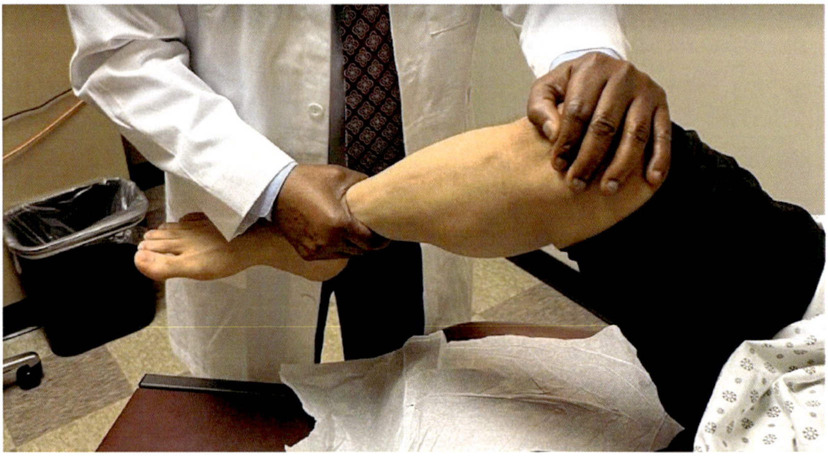

ASSESSMENT OF PATELLOFEMORAL LIGAMENT

The medial patellofemoral ligament is in the second layer of the three soft tissue layers within the medial aspect of the knee. The main function of the medial patellofemoral ligament is to provide restraint to the patella during early knee flexion (0-30 degrees).

The Patella apprehension test

1. Instruct the patient to be positioned in a supine or sitting position on the bench with his/her knee flexed to 30 degrees.
2. The quadriceps should be relaxed to allow passive movements of the patella.
3. Use your thumb of both hands and press them on the medial side of the patient's patella.
4. The test is positive if it produces pain and apprehension. If the test is positive, take notice of the patient's facial expression, as he/she may be surprised by the amount of lateral displacement of the patella, and may feel uncomfortable or apprehensive, as the patella reaches the maximal lateral displacement

PATELLAR REFLEX (KNEE JERK)

1. Strike the reflex hammer on the patellar tendon located just below the inferior pole of the patella and just above the tibial tubercle.
2. Hold firmly the thigh with your free hand to feel contraction of the quadriceps muscle and observe simultaneous extension of the lower leg at the knee.
3. Repeat the technique for the other leg.

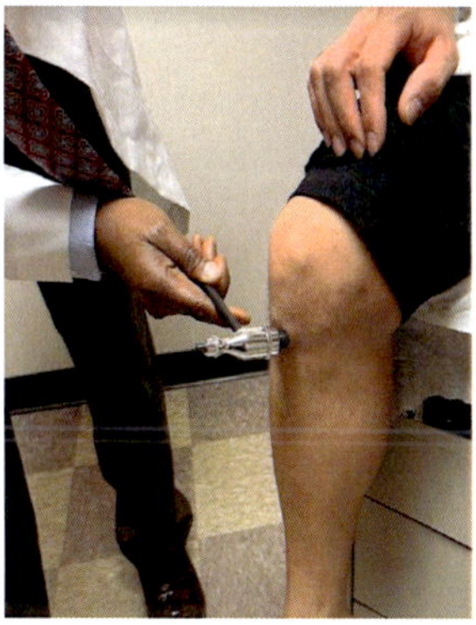

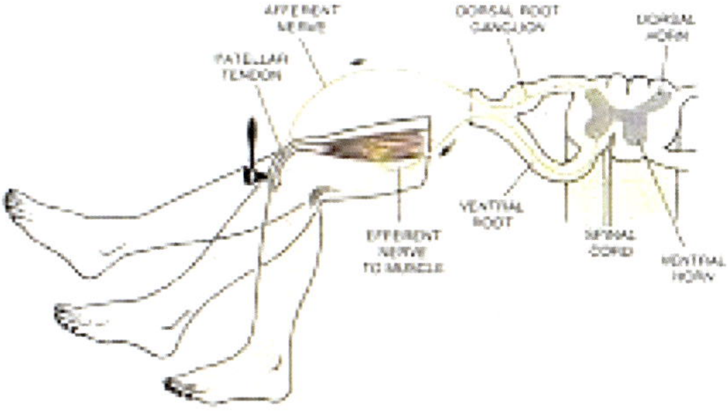

COMPLETION OF THE KNEE EXAMS

The examination of the knee is completed by:

1. Palpation of the Popliteal artery
2. Assessment of Sensory component of the Neuro exam- Light (superficial touch), and temperature as already described in the Neuro exam component

EXAMINATION OF ANKLE AND FOOT

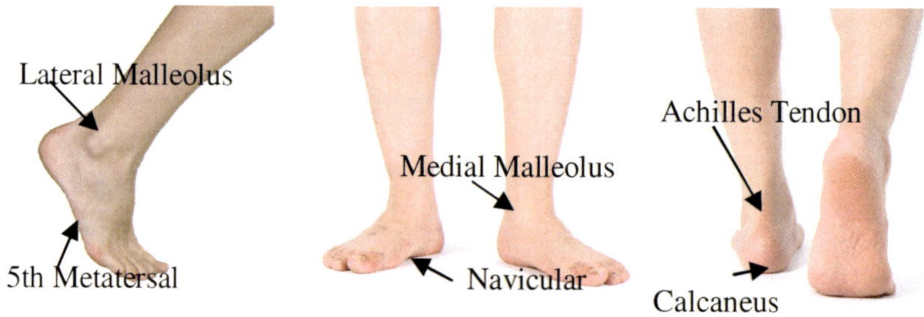

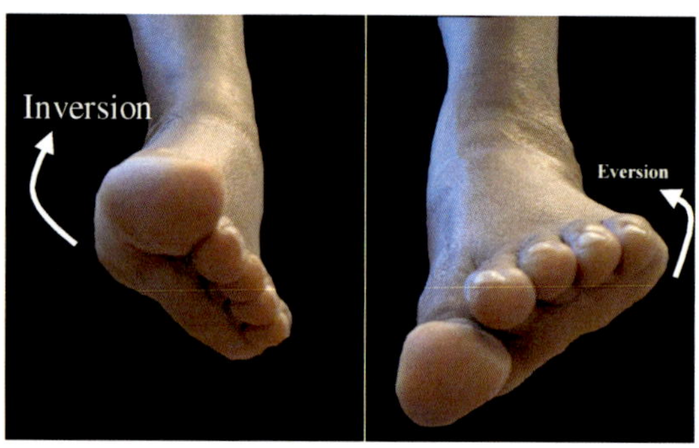

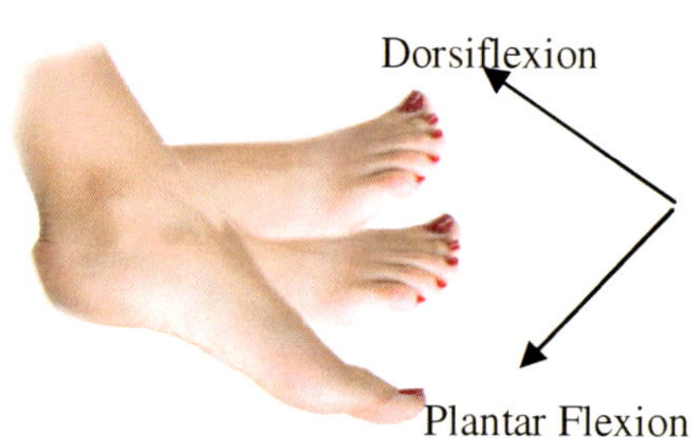

1. Instruct patient to stand.
2. Instruct patient to walk and examine the gait.
3. Inspect the ankles and feet for swelling and deformities. Note any abnormal foot anatomy (e.g., clawfoot, flatfoot, and hallux valgus).
4. Seat patient with feet dangling off the side of the examination table.
5. Palpate the medial and lateral malleoli.
6. Palpate the body of the Achilles tendon and its insertion.
7. Test PROM (Passive Range of Motion) of the ankle by dorsiflexion (normal range is 0 to 20 degrees), inversion (normal range is 0 to 35 degrees), eversion (normal range 0 to 15 degrees), plantar flexion (normal range is 0 to 50 degrees) and the subtalar joint.
8. Instruct patient to flex the toes (curl up your toes as tight as you can) and extend (extend your toes backwards, like you're trying to point them towards your head.) the toes.
9. Instruct patient to perform AROM (Active Range of Motion) by dorsiflexion, plantar flexion, eversion and inversion against resistant (this is testing the subtalar joint actively).
10. Palpate the forefoot: grasp the metatarsophalangeal joints by placing thumb and index fingers across the forefoot and attempt to compress the forefoot.
11. Also remember pain in the first metatarsophalangeal joint associated with redness and swelling may suggest a condition termed podagra, which is associated with gout.
12. Palpate the Proximal Interphalangeal (PIP) and Distal Interphalangeal (DIP) joints. If pain is elicited, it may indicate an early sign of rheumatoid arthritis or a fracture.

ACHILLES REFLEX

1. Place the foot to be examined in dorsiflexion.
2. Strike the Achilles tendon just above its insertion on the posterior aspect of the calcaneus. A (+) positive response is a mild plantar flexion.

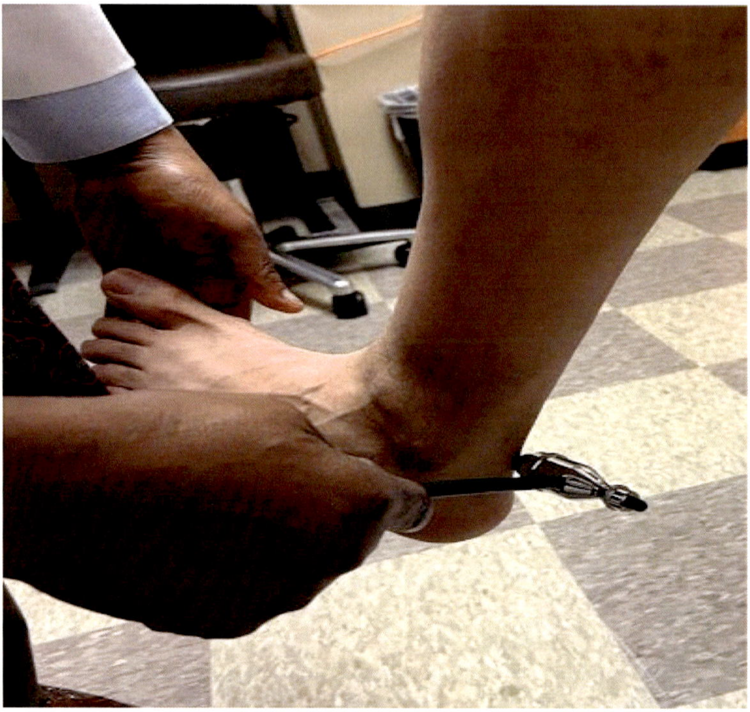

COMPLETION OF THE FOOT AND ANKLE EXAMINATION

1. Palpation of the Dorsalis Pedis and Posterior Tibial artery.
2. Assessing for Babinski reflex, ankle clonus, joint position sense, vibration, and the sensory component as already itemized on the neuro component of this manual.

SKILL ASSESSMENTS

SKILL ASSESSMENT: ABDOMEN EXAMINATION

	Introduction	Completed (+1)	Not Completed (-1)	Completed Incorrectly (-1)
1.	Student introduced self			
2.	Student washed hands			
3.	Student explained the examination to the patient			
4.	Student had patient lie flat, ensured patient's hands to the side, and table extension is out.			

	Inspection	Completed (+1)	Not Completed (-1)	Completed Incorrectly (-1)
5.	Inspected the abdomen			

	Auscultation *This must be done prior to palpation or percussion or the student must REMEDIATE	Completed (+1)	Not Completed (-1)	Completed Incorrectly (-1)
6.	All four (4) quadrants			

	Percussion	Completed (+1)	Not Completed (-1)	Completed Incorrectly (-1)
7.	All four (4) Quadrants			
8.	Liver span			
9.	Spleen (student makes attempt)			

	Palpation	Completed (+1)	Not Completed (-1)	Completed Incorrectly (-1)
10.	All four (4) quadrants (light OR deep acceptable)			
11.	Liver (bimanual OR hooking method acceptable)			
12.	Spleen			
13.	Kidneys (both left & right)			
14.	Aorta (assess aortic pulsations)			
15.	Assessed rebound tenderness			
16.	Assessed for Murphy's Sign			
17.	Assessed for Costal Vertebral Angle tenderness			
18.	Student verbalized s/he would be performing a RECTAL EXAM for completeness			

PRACTICE WORKSHOP: ABDOMEN EXAMINATION

	Introduction	Completed Correctly	Omitted	Performed Incorrectly
1.	Student introduced self			
2.	Student washed hands			
3.	Student explained the examination to the patient			
4.	Student had patient lie flat, ensured patient' hands to the side and table extension is out.			

	Inspection	Completed Correctly	Omitted	Performed Incorrectly
5.	Stand on the right side of the bed with the patient in supine position, legs flat and **arms at side.**			
6.	Ensure patient's comfortable, pillow under head, chest drape and table extension is pulled out.			
7.	Drape chest, expose abdomen fully and assess patient comfort level.			
8.	Observe contour of abdomen while standing at the right side of patient.			
9.	Stand near the foot of the bed and observe symmetry of abdomen contour (have patient breath deeply).			
10.	Ask patient to lift head and shoulders off bed (check for abdominal hernia).			
11.	Observe aortic pulsation.			
12.	Inspect skin for: color, scars, lesions, striae, distention, hair distribution.			

	Auscultation	Completed Correctly	Omitted	Performed Incorrectly
13.	Assure that your stethoscope is warm.			
14.	Place stethoscope on the skin with just enough pressure to assure good contact.			
15.	Start in the right lower quad and listen to bowel sounds.			
16.	Proceed to listen in all four quads. When you hear bowel sounds assess them and move to the next area on the abdomen.			
17.	Assess and document the frequency and pitch of the sounds.			

18.	If bowel sounds **are absent** you must listen for a full 5 minutes, over the abdomen in all four quads, **before concluding and charting** that bowel sounds are not present.			
	Auscultation of Vascular Sounds	Completed Correctly	Omitted	Performed Incorrectly
	Bruits			
19.	Use the bell, pressing gently over the abdomen, starting in the epigastric region at the aorta, renal, iliac, and femoral arteries. *(These are normally silent. If a bruit is heard listen agaln to the heart. Some murmurs will radiate to the abdomen, especially those of aortic valve origin).*			
	Venous hum			
20.	Listen on or below the right costal margin.			
21.	It is softer than a bruit and continuous rather than systolic in timing.			
	Friction Rubs			
22.	Place diaphragm over each costal margin.			
23.	Have patient breath slowly and deeply (listen over the liver and spleen area). *(Normally silent, friction rubs are high pitched and associated with respiration).*			

	Percussion	Completed Correctly	Omitted	Performed Incorrectly
	Abdomen			
24.	Percuss lightly in each quadrant (Tympany usually predominates).			
25.	Percuss in all 9 areas of the abdomen. Percussion techniques may vary. A circular, continuous, horizontal or vertical technique may be used			
26.	Percuss over areas of unexpected bulging.			
	Liver (Estimate Size)			
27.	Percuss in the right midclavicular line starting in the mid chest. Percuss from area of resonance to area of dullness in 1 inch steps. Mark this point			
28.	Locate lower border by percussing upward beginning at the level of the umbilicus. Percuss from tympany to dullness in 1-inch step beginning at the level of the umbilicus.			

	Mark this Point			
29.	Measure the distance between the 2 points in the midclavicular line (6 to 12cm is normal)			
30.	If the liver seems enlarged percuss from midsternal and anterior axillary lines.			
	Spleen (Estimate Size)	**Completed Correctly**	**Omitted**	**Performed Incorrectly**
31.	The spleen lies between the 9th and 11th intercostal space posterior to the mid axillary line.			
32.	Percuss from the midline in several directions toward the area of splenic dullness (beginning at the 6th rib).			
33.	Continue to percuss over the lower intercostal space (9th through 12th). *Tympany is normal heard. If the spleen is enlarged, you will hear dullness).*			
	Gastric Bubble			
34.	Percuss the gastric air bubble horizontally and vertically in the area of the lower anterior left rib cage.			

	Light Palpation (Detect tenderness, muscular spasms or rigidity)	**Completed Correctly**	**Omitted**	**Performed Incorrectly**
35.	Warm your hands.			
36.	To aid in relaxation of the abdomen, place a pillow beneath the knees.			
37.	Palpate any area of tenderness last.			
38.	Hand and arm are parallel to the abdominal skin.			
39.	Observe patient's face for any signs of discomfort.			
40.	If stomach wall is tense, have patient flex knees.			
	Deep Palpation: (Organ size or abdomen mass) Survey abdomen for masses			
41.	Palpate with a two-handed technique.			
42.	Place one hand down on the abdomen and place the other hand over it.			
43.	Use the top hand to press down while feeling the structures with the other hand. The motion has three components: A. Push hands forward B. Push down C. Press and pull back			

44.	Palpate through each quadrant. * **Mass –** Describe and document depth, size, shape, location, consistency, and tenderness. If you cannot tell if it is in the wall or not, have the patient tense their abdomen. (Masses in the abdominal wall will remain palpable)			
	Liver Bimanual Method	**Completed Correctly**	**Omitted**	**Performed Incorrectly**
45.	Stand on the patient's right side.			
46.	Place left hand posteriorly between patient's right 12th rib and iliac crest.			
47.	Place right hand near the umbilicus, lateral to the rectus abdominus muscle. Always begin low in case the liver is enlarged.			
48.	Aim fingers vertically or obliquely to patient's upper left.			
49.	Lift left hand up slightly and press slightly in with right hand.			
50.	Have patient breath deeply and feel for the liver edge as it descends. If you do not feel the edge of the liver, bring your right hand up 1 inch and try again. (The liver edge is usually not palpable)			
51.	If you feel the edge of the liver, check for tenderness.			
52.	**Check for Murphy's sign.** A catch in the respiration is a positive finding, strongly suggestive of **Acute Cholecystitis.**			
	Liver Hooking Maneuver	**Completed Correctly**	**Omitted**	**Performed Incorrectly**
53.	Stand above the patient, facing toward feet.			
54.	Place both hands, side by side, below the right costal margin.			
55.	Ask patient to inhale deeply and curl fingertips inward and upward under the patient's rib cage.			
	Spleen			
56.	Stand to the patient's right side.			
57.	Reach with your left hand over and under the patient's left posterior inferior costal margin.			
58.	Place your right hand near the umbilicus.			
59.	With fingers aimed upward, toward the patient's spleen lift up with the left hand to displace the spleen anteriorly.			

60.	Ask the patient to breath deeply while palpating for the spleen.			
61.	If palpable, describe and document the edge in cm's below the left costal margin.			
62.	If enlarge, roll the patient to right side with knees and hips slightly flexed and try palpation again.			
	Right kidney			
63.	Place left hand under flank.			
64.	Place right hand below the right costal margin with the fingertips positioned toward the midline.			
65.	Ask patient to inhale deeply.			
66.	With left hand lift upward while right hand depresses deeply. The lower pole may be felt as a smooth rounded mass as it descends during inspiration.			
	Left kidney	**Completed Correctly**	**Omitted**	**Performed Incorrectly**
67.	Remain on the patient's right side.			
68.	Reach with left hand over and under patient's left posterior inferior costal margin.			
69.	Place right hand near the umbilicus aiming fingertips more toward the left flank.			
70.	Ask patient to inhale deeply.			
71.	With left hand lift upward while right hand depresses deeply. The lower pole may be felt as a smooth rounded mass as it descends during inspiration.			
	Aorta			
72.	Press the fingertips of the right hand deeply but gently into the epigastric area slightly left of the midline.			
73.	Gauge the width of the pulsation.			
74.	Encircling with thumb and fingers, and press gently.			
75.	Describe and document the aorta pulsation (aorta is 2.5 to 4cm wide). *Note: Alternate technique for obese individual; using both hands press fingertips deeply in on both sided of the aortic pulsation.*			
	Rebound tenderness			

76.	Hold hand 90 degrees to the abdomen and press the fingertips firmly, but slowly, into the abdomen near the area of suspicion or pain.			
77.	***Release quickly*** (IF there is **rebound tenderness,** there will be pain upon release of your hand. Have the patient point to the pain).			
78.	**Rovsing's sign:** Press in the left lower quadrant. Sudden release will cause pain in the right lower quadrant (Indicative of appendicitis).			
79.	**McBurney's Point:** tenderness in the right lower quadrant is a sign of localized peritoneal irritation.			
	Additional Tests	**Completed Correctly**	**Omitted**	**Performed Incorrectly**
	Ascites (Percussion or Palpation)			
	Shifting Dullness			
80.	Percuss from the umbilical area downward toward the flank in several direction horizon to the mid line.			
81.	To map the lateral borders, note the change from tympany to dullness.			
82.	Roll patient onto one side; percuss and identify the border again.			
	Fluid Wave			
83.	Ask patient to place ulnar edge of hand down into the midline of abdomen.			
84.	Place one hand on either flank.			
85.	Tap the other flank sharply with the other hand. (with ascities, you will feel a fluid wave against the other hand)			
	Hyperesthesia (Peritoneal Inflammation)			
86.	Gently pull skin together and lift a fold.			
87.	Stroke the skin with an object lightly.			
	Obturator sign (*For Deeper Inflammation)			
88.	Flex the right knee and hip 90 degrees (upon the chest).			
89.	Grasp the ankle and rotate the hip internally and externally.			
90.	Intrapelvic inflammation will cause lower-quadrant pain on the affected side. This discomfort indicates a positive test result.			

	Psoas (Iliopsoas) sign			
91.	Ask patient to raise a straightened right leg against resistance.			
92.	Alternatively, ask patient to lie on left side and the examiner gently hyperextends straightened leg to stretch the psoas major muscle.			
	Renal Tenderness			
93.	Place patient in sitting position.			
94.	Place fingers over the costovertebral angle and lightly palpate. If no pain place left palm over one costovertebral angle.			
95.	Percuss lightly.			
96.	Percuss firmly with right fist. (Check each side)			
	Rectal Exam			
97.	A rectal exam should **ALWAYS** complete an abdominal complaint.			

PRACTICE WORKSHOP: CARDIOVASCULAR EXAM

	Introduction	Completed Correctly	Omitted	Performed Incorrectly
1.	Student introduced self			
2.	Student washed hands			
3.	Student explained the examination to the patient			

	Examination of the Neck Veins (ALL cardiac examinations begin with examination of the neck veins)	Completed Correctly	Omitted	Performed Incorrectly
	Inspection			
4.	Explain to patient what you will be doing.			
5.	Position patient supine with head of exam table elevated at a 30 - 45° angle. **Remove any pillow to avoid flexing the neck.**			
6.	Have patient turn head contralateral to side being examined with the neck in the same plane as the thorax, (use tangential lighting to increase shadows).			
7.	Locate the sternal angle, a horizontal ridge within 5cm of the sternal notch.			
8.	Inspect the *external jugular vein(JV)* which appears as a slightly distended column above the right clavicle, showing a small up-and down oscillation. The *internal JV* is located beneath the stern mastoid muscle. Pulsations transmit to the skin are often seen as a rhythmic movement at the base of the muscle.			
9.	Observe the pulsation at the base of the stern mastoid.			
10.	While auscultating the heart with the bell or diaphragm at the PMI **(not over clothes)** observe for the *venous pulsation.*			
11.	Inspect hands and nail beds for peripheral circulation.			

	Auscultation of the Carotid Artery	Completed Correctly	Omitted	Performed Incorrectly
12.	Lightly place bell of stethoscope over EACH carotid artery (may use diaphragm also).			
13.	Listen, while patient hold holds breath, for bruits, or a transmitted murmur. **Note: if no bruits are appreciated proceed to palpate the carotid arteries.**			

	Palpation of the Carotid Artery	Completed Correctly	Omitted	Performed Incorrectly
14.	Turn patient's head slightly toward the side being examined.			
15.	Place the tip of one or two fingers between the trachea and, stern mastoid muscle.			
16.	**Palpate one side at a time.**			
17.	Note rate, rhythm and intensity.			
18.	Note any palpable vibration.			
19.	Palpate the other carotid artery.			

	Measurement	Completed Correctly	Omitted	Performed Incorrectly
20.	Locate the highest level of pulsation in the internal JV, if not visible tangential lighting may be used to better discriminate the level of pulsation. The external JV may also be used when the internal JV is not appreciated.			
21.	If the oscillating level of distention is located above the sternal angle, hold a horizontal marker from the top of the visible oscillating level of distention over to and above the manubriosternal angle. *Place the ruler vertically on the sternal angle and read **up** to the level of the marker.*			
22.	Measure the vertical distance from the highest level of pulsation to the manubriosternal angle (Angle of Louis).			
23.	Record the distance in centimeters above or below the sternal angle **and angle of inclination.**			

	Palpation of Pulses	Completed Correctly	Omitted	Performed Incorrectly
24.	Palpate the patient's temporal artery bilaterally with the pads of your fingers. *(note rate, rhythm and intensity and any presence of tenderness)*			
25.	Have patient clinch teeth to palpate the temporalis muscle. *(Tenderness in the geriatric population **MAY** indicate temporal arteritis)*			
26.	Palpate brachial pulse by grasping the biceps brachialis muscle belly elevating it with the fingers finding the pulse. The			

	brachial artery may be felt medially just under the belly, or palpated just medial to the tendinous insertion of the biceps muscle. Stand in from of patient and palpate both brachial arteries simultaneously.			
27.	Palpate the radial pulse with finger pads of the index and third finger. (Note rate, rhythm and intensity).			
28.	Palpate the femoral pulse in the groin region (Note rate, rhythm and intensity).			
29.	Palpate the dorsalis pedis artery bilaterally with some dorsiflexion of the foot.			
30.	Palpate the posterior tibial artery with slight plantar flexion of the foot. Both arteries may be evaluated simultaneously. ***Remember the posterior tibial pulses can be absent in 15% of normal young subject; however, it is the most sensitive sign of occlusive peripheral arterial disease in patients over the age of 60 years when it is not palpable.***			

	Examination of the PMI	Completed Correctly	Omitted	Performed Incorrectly
31.	Place the patient in supine position.			
32.	Stand at the right side of the patient.			
33.	Shine light tangentially onto the left side of the chest, 5th intercostal space, mid-clavicular line.			
34.	Observe for movement above the apex medially.			
35.	Describe and document the size and location of the impulse.			

	Palpation of PMI	Completed Correctly	Omitted	Performed Incorrectly
36.	Palpate the apical impulse placing the fingertips on the chest in the left fifth intercostal space (ICS), midclavicular line (MCL). The PMI is usually within 10cm of the midsternal line and normally 2-3cm in diameter. (approximately)			
37.	If the PMI is not palpable, move fingertips medial or lateral in the area of the cardiac apex.			
38.	Place index fingertip on interspace above and ring finger on interspace below the apical impulse; rest hand flat and assess the impulse.			

39.	Describe and document the size, intensity, location, and duration.			

	Examination of the Precordium (Inspection)	Completed Correctly	Omitted	Performed Incorrectly
40.	Inspect the precordium for color, scars, lesions, striae, lifts, chest configuration, and use of accessory muscles with respiration.			
	Examination of the Precordium (Palpation)			
41.	Palpate over the entire precordium for impulse or vibratory thrills. Palpate in order: ▪ Sternoclavicular area ▪ Second right interspace and sternal border ▪ Second left interspace and sternal border ▪ Left lower sternal border ▪ Apical area			
42.	Slip the fingertips under the right costal margin near the xyphoid process. Palpate for right ventricular enlargement.			

	Percussion	Completed Correctly	Omitted	Performed Incorrectly
43.	Use percussion to outline the left lateral heart border.			
44.	Percuss in 1" intervals from anterior axillary line to sternum; in the third, fourth, and fifth intercostal spaces. It is best to have patient hold breath mid-expiration because the heart moves with respirations.			
45.	The three points will form a line. Measure this border directly from the mid-sternum. Normally, during percussion you can determine a change from resonance to dullness about 6cm laterally to the left of the sternum. A comparison of measurement can be directly related to posterior – anterior chest roentgenogram.			

	Auscultation of the Precordium	Completed Correctly	Omitted	Performed Incorrectly
46.	Place the diaphragm firmly over the apex and listen for S1 and S2.			
47.	Listen for rate, rhythm, intensity and splitting of S1 and S2.			
48.	While the patient is supine ausculatate the Aortic, Pulmonic, Tricuspid and Mitral valve area with the diaphragm and then bell. *This should be in a Z pattern.*			
49.	Listen attentively for extra heart sounds and murmurs in systole and diastole.			
50.	Position patient in left lateral decubitus and listen over the apex with the **bell.**			
51.	Sit patient up and listen with the **diaphragm** and **bell** in all four auscultation areas again.			
52.	Have patient lean slightly forward and listen over the base of the heart with the diaphragm.			
53.	Have patient fully exhale and hold breath. Listen at the base of the heart (2nd intercostal space) and the right and left sternal border of the heart (3rd and 4th intercostal space). Listen for aortic insufficiency murmurs.			
54.	Describe and document findings. Note: **Murmur** – if heart record the following characteristics: ▪ Timing in the cardiac cycle ▪ Location ▪ Radiation ▪ Duration ▪ Intensity ▪ Pitch ▪ Quality ▪ Relationship to respiration ▪ Relationship to body position			

PRACTICE WORKSHOP: EYE EXAM

	Introduction	Completed (+1)	Not Completed (-1)	Completed Incorrectly (-1)
1.	Student introduced self			
2.	Student washed hands			
3.	Student explained the examination to the patient			

	Examined the External Adnexa	Completed (+1)	Not Completed (-1)	Completed Incorrectly (-1)
4.	Lids			
5.	Lashes			
6.	Lacrimal			
7.	Lymphatics			

	Examined the Internal Structures	Completed (+1)	Not Completed (-1)	Completed Incorrectly (-1)
8.	Sclera			
9.	Cornea			
10.	Iris			
11.	Pupils			
12.	Anterior Chamber (viewed from one side)			

	Visual	Completed (+1)	Not Completed (-1)	Completed Incorrectly (-1)
13.	Student assessed Visual Acuity (Snellen or Rosenbaum card)			
14.	Student assessed the Pupillary Light Reflex (direct and consensual)			
15.	Student assessed Extraocular Muscles **(H pattern)**			
16.	Student assessed Convergence			
17.	Student performed Cover Test			
18.	Student assessed Visual Fields (by Confrontation)			

SKILL ASSESSMENT: HEAD, EARS, NOSE, THROAT EXAMINATION

	Introduction	Completed (+1)	Not Completed (-1)	Completed Incorrectly
1.	Student Introduced self			
2.	Student washed hands			
3.	Student explained the examination to the patient			

	Examination of the Head	Completed (+1)	Not Completed (-1)	Completed Incorrectly
4.	Inspected the hair			
5.	Inspected the eyes			
6.	Inspected the neck			
7.	Palpated the scalp			

	Examination of the Neck	Completed (+1)	Not Completed (-1)	Completed Incorrectly
8.	Palpated the occipital nodes			
9.	Palpated the anterior auricular nodes			
10.	Palpated the posterior auricular nodes			
11.	Palpated the posterior cervical nodes			
12.	Palpated the superficial cervical nodes			
13.	Palpated the deep cervical nodes			
14.	Palpated the tonsillar nodes			
15.	Palpated the submandibular nodes			
16.	Palpated the submental nodes			
17.	Palpate the supraclavicular nodes			

	Examination of the Ears	Completed (+1)	Not Completed (-1)	Completed Incorrectly (-1)
18.	Examined the external ear			
19.	Performed the Whisper Test			
20.	Performed the Rinne test			
21.	Performed the Weber test			
22.	Performed the otosopic examination			

	Examination of the Nose	Completed (+1)	Not Completed (-1)	Completed Incorrectly (-1)
23.	Inspected the nose externally			
24.	Palpated the sinuses			
25.	Examined the internal nasal passages			
26.	Transilluminated the frontal sinuses			
27.	Tranilluminated the maxillary sinuses			

	Examination of Pharynx & Oral Cavity	Completed (+1)	Not Completed (-1)	Completed Incorrectly (-1)
28.	Used a light to inspect the pharynx			
29.	Used a tongue depressor to inspect the pharynx			
30.	Inspected the lips			
31.	Inspected the lips			
32.	Inspected the buccal mucosa			
33.	Inspected the teeth			
34.	Inspected the palate			
35.	Inspected the tongue			
36.	Inspected the floor of the mouth			

SKILL ASSESSMENT: HEART EXAMINATION

	Introduction	Completed (+1)	Not Completed	Completed Incorrectly (-1)
1.	Student introduced self			
2.	Student washed hands			
3.	Student explained the examination to the patient			

	Examination of the Neck and Arteries	Completed (+1)	Not Completed	Completed Incorrectly (-1)
4.	Ask patient to hold breath			
5.	Auscultated (listened) to left & right carotid arteries			
6.	Palpated left & right carotid arteries (one at a time)			
7.	Inspected for the JVP at 30° angle			
8.	Measured the JVP at 30° angle			

	Inspection & Palpation Pulses	Completed (+1)	Not Completed	Completed Incorrectly (-1)
9.	Inspected hands & nail beds for peripheral circulation			
10.	Palpated the temporal artery			
11.	Palpated for radial pulse			
12.	Palpated the femoral pulse			
13.	Palpated dorsalis pedis and posterior tibial pulse			

	Inspection & Palpation of Heart	Completed (+1)	Not Completed	Completed Incorrectly (-1)
14.	Inspected the PMI			
15.	Palpated the PMI			
16.	Palpated the precordium of impules/thrills			

	Auscultation of Heart Listened in SUPINE position with BELL	Completed (+1)	Not Completed	Completed Incorrectly (-1)
17.	Aortic			
18.	Pulmonic			
19.	Tricuspid			
20.	Mitral			
21.	Left lateral decubitus position (apex only)			

	Auscultation of Heart **Listened in SUPINE position with DIAPHRAGM**	**Completed (+1)**	**Not Completed (-1)**	**Performed Incorrectly (-1)**
22.	Aortic			
23.	Pulmonic			
24.	Tricuspid			
25.	Mitral			

	Auscultation of Heart **Listened to in an UPRIGHT (Sitting) position with DIAPHRAGM**	**Completed (+1)**	**Not Completed (-1)**	**Performed Incorrectly (-1)**
26.	Aortic			
27.	Pulmonic			
28.	Tricuspid			
29.	Mitral			

	Auscultation of Heart **Listened to in an UPRIGHT (Sitting) position with DIAPHRAGM**	**Completed (+1)**	**Not Completed (-1)**	**Performed Incorrectly (-1)**
30.	Aortic			
31.	Pulmonic			
32.	Tricuspid			
33.	Mitral			
34.	Leaning-forward (exhales and holds breath) Listens at BASE of heart 2nd intercostal space			
35.	Leaning-forward (exhales and holds breath) Listens at RIGHT sternal border of heart 3rd and 4th intercostal space			
36.	Leaning-forward (exhales and holds breath) Listens at LEFT sternal border of heart 3rd and 4th intercostal space			

PRACTICE WORKSHOP: LUNG EXAM

	Introduction	Completed (+1)	Not Completed (-1)	Completed Incorrectly (-1)
1.	Student introduced sell			
2.	Student washed hands			
3.	Student explained the examination to the patient			

	Inspection	Completed (+1)	Not Completed (-1)	Completed Incorrectly (-1)
4.	Inspected the face and lips (discoloration, etc.)			
5.	Inspected patient's posture			
6.	Inspected neck, accessory muscles, JVD			
7.	Inspected for chest wall deformity			
8.	Respiratory rate, pattern, and depth of breathing			
9.	Inspected hand (clubbing, discoloration)			

	Palpation	Completed (+1)	Not Completed (-1)	Completed Incorrectly (-1)
10.	Palpated for masses and tenderness			
11.	Palpated tracheal position			
12.	Performed chest excursion (posterior)			

	Tacile Fremitus – POSTERIOR ONLY	Completed (+1)	Not Completed (-1)	Completed Incorrectly (-1)
13.	Student used ulnar, fingertips or palm of hand.			
14.	Student used across-down pattern			
15.	Assessed **6** locations (3 left & 3 right) posteriorly (above, between & below scapula)			
16.	Assessed diaphragmatic excursion			

	Percussion	Completed (+1)	Not Completed (-1)	Completed Incorrectly (-1)
17.	Student used across-down pattern (both anteriorly and posteriorly)			
18.	Percussed to **8** locations (4 left & right) anteriorly (apices, 1st, 2nd and 5th spaces)			
19.	Percussed **6** location (3 left & 3 right) posteriorly (above, between & below scapula)			

	Auscultation	Completed (+1)	Not Completed (-1)	Completed Incorrectly (-1)
20.	Student used across-down pattern (both anteriorly and posteriorly)			
21.	Listened to **8** locations (4 left & 4 right) anteriorly (apices, 1st, 2nd and 5th spaces)			
22.	Listened to **6** locations (3 left & 3 right) posteriorly (above, between & below scapula)			
23.	Performs Bronchophony (1 area vs all over)			
24.	Performs Whisper pectoriloquy (1 area vs all over)			
25.	Perform Egophony (1 area vs all over)			

SKILL ASSESSMENT SESSION: MEDICAL HISTORY INTERVIEW

	INTRODUCTION	Completed	Not Completed
1.	Student introduced self		
2.	Student washed hands		
3.	Student explained the reason for encounter		
4.	Student asked patient how they would like to be addressed		

	GENERAL HISTORY	Completed	Not Completed
5.	Age		
6.	Date of Birth		
7.	Place of Birth		

	CHIEF COMPLAINT	Completed	Not Completed
8.	Did student elicit chief complaint		

	HISTORY OF PARENT ILLNESS	Completed	Not Completed
9.	Chief Complaint appropriately detailed		
10.	7 dimensions of cardinal symptom (quality, quality, location, setting, chronology, aggravating/alleviating, associated symptoms)		
11.	Chronological and well organized		
12.	Incorporates elements of PMH, FH, SH		
13.	Pertinent ROS (positive and negative)		

	PAST MEDICAL HISTORY	Completed	Not Completed
14.	Sufficient detail of diagnosis, onset, complications and therapy/treatment		
15.	Gynecologic History		
16.	Obstetric history		

	PAST SURGICAL HISTORY	Completed	Not Completed
17.	Procedure, date of procedure, surgeon and location		

	MEDICATION	Completed	Not Completed
18.	Prescribed: dose, route, frequency		
19.	Over the counter		
20.	Herbal		

	ALLERGIES	Completed	Not Completed
21.	Medication: Type of reaction		
22.	Seasonal		

	SOCAL HISTORY	Completed	Not Completed
23.	Occupation		
24.	Marital status		
25.	Education		
26.	Tobacco use		
27.	Alcohol use		
28.	Substance abuse		
29.	Functional status (exercise, diet)		
30.	Living situation		
31.	Sexual history		

	FAMILY HISTORY	Completed	Not Completed
33.	State of health of first degree relatives		
34.	Common hereditary conditions addressed (CAD, CA, DM, RTOH)		

	REVIEW OF SYSTEMS	Completed	Not Completed
34.	Positive findings addressed with adequate depth		
35.	Does not include PMH		
36.	Pertinent negative findings addressed		

PRACTICE WORKSHOP: MUSCULOSKELETAL SYSTEM EXAM

	Introduction	Completed (+1)	Not Completed (-1)	Performed Incorrectly (-1)
1.	Student introduced self.			
2.	Student washed hands.			
3.	Student explained the examination to the patient.			

	Temporal Mandibular Joint (TMJ)	Completed (+1)	Not Completed (-1)	Performed Incorrectly (-1)
4.	Palpated TMJ			

	Neck Pulse Examination	Completed (+1)	Not Completed (-1)	Performed Incorrectly (-1)
5.	Inspected cervical region.			
6.	Palpated spinous processes.			
7.	Palpated paraspinal musculature.			
8.	Examined cervical flexion.			
9.	Examined cervical extension.			
10.	Examined cervical rotation.			
11.	Examined side flexion.			

	Shoulders (Not Over Clothes)	Completed (+1)	Not Completed (-1)	Performed Incorrectly (-1)
12.	Inspected for symmetry and deformities			
13.	Palpated shoulder, acromioclavicular, sternoclavicular, and costosternal joints.			
14.	Performed AROM (active range of motion).			

	Elbow	Completed (+1)	Not Completed (-1)	Performed Incorrectly (-1)
15.	Inspection for deformities and swelling.			
16.	Examined for flexion and extension against resistance.			
17.	Palpated medial and lateral epicondyles.			
18.	Palpated.			

	Hand	Completed (+1)	Not Completed (-1)	Performed Incorrectly (-1)
19.	Inspected nail beds, finger pads, and thenar/hypothenar musculature			
20.	Checked for sensory deficits in median / ulnar/radial nerve distribution			
21.	Palpated metacarpophalangeal joints			
22.	Wrist Flexion			
23.	Examined wrist extension.			
24.	Examined thumb opposition.			
25.	Examined hand intrinsic by squeezing fingers together against resistance.			

	Thoracolumbar spine	Completed (+1)	Not Completed (-1)	Performed Incorrectly (-1)
26.	Inspected back (noting curvature and deformities).			
27.	Palpated thoracic and lumbar spinous processes.			
28.	Palpated paraspinal musculature.			
29.	Examined flexion.			
30.	Examined side flexion.			
31.	Examined rotation.			
32.	Performed straight leg raise (only one leg).			

	Hip/Gluteal region	Completed (+1)	Not Completed (-1)	Performed Incorrectly (-1)
33.	Inspected gluteal region for pressure ulcers.			
34.	Palpated hip and sub trochanteric bursa.			

	Leg/Knee	Completed (+1)	Not Completed (-1)	Performed Incorrectly (-1)
35.	Inspected legs for venous stasis, edema or vessel abnormalities.			
36.	Inspected knee for joint effusion and deformities.			
37.	Palpated in the popliteal fossa.			
38.	Palpated the patella and joint line.			
39.	Examined flexion and extension against resistance.			
40.	Positioned themselves in proper position for the anterior drawer test.			

	Ankle/Foot	Completed (+1)	Not Completed (-1)	Performed Incorrectly (-1)
41.	Inspected foot for abnormalities.			
42.	Palpated malleoli.			
43.	Palpated heel and insertion of Achilles tendon.			
44.	Palpated the metatarsophalangeal joints.			
45.	Palpated planter / dorsiflexion against resistance.			
46.	Palpated inversion / eversion against resistance.			

	Reflexes	Completed (+1)	Not Completed (-1)	Performed Incorrectly (-1)
47.	Examined the biceps brachi reflex. (C5, C6)			
48.	Examined the triceps reflex. (C6, C7, C8)			
49.	Examined the patellar reflex. (L3, L4)			
50.	Examined the ankle jerk reflex. (S1)			

PRACTICE WORKSHOP: NEUROLOGICAL & MMSE EXAMINATION

	Introduction	Completed (+1)	Not Completed (-1)	Performed I Incorrectly (-1)
1.	Student introduced self			
2.	Student washed hands			
3.	Student explained the examination to the patient			

Mini-Mental Status Exam

	Orientation	Completed (+1)	Not Completed (-1)	Performed I Incorrectly (-1)
4.	Name this hospital or building. (Meharry)			
5.	What floor of the building are you on?			
6.	What country or country is this?			
7.	What state are you in?			
8.	What city (or town) are you in now?			
9.	What year is it?			
10.	What is the moth is it?			
11.	What is the date today?			
12.	What day of the week is it?			
13.	What season of the year is it?			

	Registration	Completed (+1)	Not Completed (-1)	Performed I Incorrectly (-1)
14.	Student named three objects and had patient repeat them.			
15.	Student asked patient to spell W-O-R-L-D backwards.			

	Recall	Completed (+1)	Not Completed (-1)	Performed I Incorrectly (-1)
16.	Student asked patient to recall and name three objects.			

	Language Tests	Completed (+1)	Not Completed (-1)	Performed I Incorrectly (-1)
17.	Asked patient to identify an object she/he pointed to. Example: watch, pen Repeated a phrase: "No its, ands, or buts"			
18.	Repeated a phrase: "No its, ands, or buts"			
19.	Gave patient a three-stage command. Example: pick up paper in right hand, fold in half, place paper on floor			
20.	Asked patient to read and perform a task. Example: close your eyes			
21.	Asked patient to write any sentence.			

	Construction	Completed (+1)	Not Completed (-1)	Performed I Incorrectly (-1)
22.	Asked patent to copy a design.			

Cranial Nerves Exam

	Cranial Nerve I	Completed (+1)	Not Completed (-1)	Performed I Incorrectly (-1)
23.	Student asked if there have been any changes in patient's smell or taste. Optional: Student may have SAFE substance for patient to smell.			

	Cranial Nerve II	Completed (+1)	Not Completed (-1)	Performed I Incorrectly (-1)
24.	Student asked patient to cover RIGHT eye with palm of hand and read Rosendbaum chart			
25.	Student asked patient to cover **LEFT eye** with palm of hand and read Rosenbaum chart			
26.	Student evaluated cardinal positions of gaze **(H pattern)**			
27.	Asked patient to look at his/her nose and not to move eyes.			

	Cranial Nerve III, IV, VI	Completed (+1)	Not Completed (-1)	Performed I Incorrectly (-1)
28.	Student evaluated cardinal positions of gaze **(H pattern)**			
29.	Asked patient to focus on a distant object (wall) then focus on a near object (pencil 5-12" in front of face)			
30.	Student performed Cover Test			

	Cranial Nerve V	Completed (+1)	Not Completed (-1)	Performed I Incorrectly (-1)
31.	**Attempted** to elicit corneal reflex			
32.	Asked patient to close eyes			
33.	Asked patient to say if she/he felt dull or sharp touch.			
34.	Checked at these locations: forehead, cheek and jaw on **RIGHT side**			
35.	Checked at these location: forehead, cheek and jaw on **LEFT side**			
36.	Asked patient to bite down			

	Cranial Nerve VII	Completed (+1)	Not Completed (-1)	Performed I Incorrectly (-1)
37.	Student asked patient to smile, puff out cheeks or show teeth.			
38.	Student asked patient to raise eyebrows or frown.			
39.	Asked patient to close eyes tight and show resistance as an attempt is made by the student to open them.			

	Cranial Nerve VIII	Completed (+1)	Not Completed (-1)	Performed I Incorrectly (-1)
40.	Performed the Rinne Test on **RIGHT ear** (tuning fork behind & beside ear)			
41.	Performed the Rinne Test on **LEFT ear** (tuning fork behind & beside ear)			
42.	Perform the Weber Test (tuning fork in middle of forehead)			

	Cranial Nerves IX and X	Completed (+1)	Not Completed (-1)	Performed I Incorrectly (-1)
43.	Student observed patient's palate as she/he said "ahh". **Attempted** to elicit Gag reflex			

	Cranial Nerve XI and XII	Completed (+1)	Not Completed (-1)	Performed I Incorrectly (-1)
44.	Student asked patient to resist motion against **RIGHT jaw.**			
45.	Student asked patient to resist motion against **LEFT jaw.**			
46.	Student asked patient to shrug and resist he/his downward motion.			
47.	Student asked patient to protrude tongue. (Observing midline)			

	Reflexes	Completed (+1)	Not Completed (-1)	Performed I Incorrectly (-1)
48.	Examined the biceps brachi reflex. (C5, C6)			
49.	Examined the triceps reflex. (C6, C7, C8)			
50.	Examined brachioradialis tendon reflex			
51.	Examined the patellar reflex. (L3, L4)			
52.	Examined the ankle jerk reflex. (S1)			

PRACTICE WORKSHOP: PULMONARY EXAM

	Introduction	Completed Correctly	Omitted	Performed Incorrectly
1.	Student introduced self			
2.	Student washed hands			
3.	Student explained the examination to the patient			

	General Inspection	Completed Correctly	Omitted	Performed Incorrectly
4.	Stand on the right side of the patient. The patient should be seated with arms folded in lap.			
5.	Observes for signs of pulmonary/respiratory distress. **(Not over clothing)** ▪ Facial: Anxiousness, restlessness, drowsiness, flushing, cyanosis, pursed lips. ▪ Neck: JVD, accessory muscle use, trachea deviation. ▪ Hands: Cyanosis and clubbing. ▪ Chest: Inspect skin anteriorly, laterally and posteriorly. Inspect the configuration of the chest (Kyphosis "barrel chest"), assess respiratory rate, depth and pattern, note any audible breathing. ▪ Postural positioning			

	Palpation (Anterior)			
6.	**Trachea**			
7.	Gently slip your thumb and index finger on each side of the trachea. Have the patient inspire deeply to check for tracheal deviation. The trachea should descend slightly in the midline.			
8.	**Chest**			
9.	Palpate the chest wall anteriorly and laterally.			

10.	Palpate firmly with your fingers for areas of tenderness.			
11.	**Tactile (vocal) Fremitus**			
12.	Press firmly onto the skin with the base of the fingers or the ulnar side of the hand. Another method of evaluating tactile fremitus is to use the fingertips. Have the patient say "ninety-nine" each time you touch the anterior chest. Start at the apex of each lung working in **across and down pattern** comparing each side of the thorax for symmetry of finding. Stay in the midclavicular lines (MCLs).			

	Percussion (Anterior)	Completed Correctly	Omitted	Performed Incorrectly
13.	Begin anteriorly ▪ Percuss the apices. ▪ Place a thumb over the right apex and strike the thumbnail. ▪ Place finger on the left apice and strike the nail. ▪ **Percuss 8 key locations:** Starting over the apices, move down the MCL percussing at the 1st, 2nd & 5th intercostal spaces or until dullness is reached using the across and down pattern descending in 2-inch steps.			
14.	Percuss laterally ▪ Percuss high in the midaxillary line, moving downward in 2-inch step until dullness is reached.			

	Auscultation (Anterior)	Completed Correctly	Omitted	Performed Incorrectly
15.	Ask patient to breathe in deeply through their mouth and exhale with their mouth open.			
16.	Auscultate with the diaphragm using the across and down pattern.			
17.	**Auscultate 8 key locations:** Starting over the apices, move down the MCL. Listening at the 1st, 2nd, and 5th intercostal spaces during a full inspiration and expiration.			
18.	Auscultate laterally down the midaxillary line in 2-inch steps.			

	Palpation (Posterior) **NOT OVER CLOTHINGS**	Completed Correctly	Omitted	Performed Incorrectly
19.	Palpate the entire posterior thorax especially where area of tenderness is found.			
20.	Evaluate for Tactile (vocal) fremitus ▪ Have patient fold arms in front. ▪ Press firmly onto the skin with base of the fingers or the ulnar side of the hand. Have patient say "ninety-nine" each time you touch the posterior chest. Start at the apex of each lung working in a **across and down pattern** comparing each side of the thorax for symmetry of finding. ▪ Avoid the scapula and spinal processes.			
21.	Evaluate posterior chest excursion. ▪ Place hands flat against the patient's back with the thumbs parallel to the midline approximately at the tenth rib. Move thumb inward medially tenting up a small fold of skin. ▪ Ask patient to inspire deeply and allow the thumbs to move apart observing symmetry. ***NOTE:*** *Additional locations can be assessed depending upon suspected problems. i.e. at the apices anteriorly and the costal margin.*			

		Completed Correctly	Omitted	Performed Incorrectly
22.	Percuss posterior thorax in at least **6 locations** (apices, above and below the scapula). ▪ Have patient fold arms to retract the scapulars. ▪ Percuss the apices above each medial scapular border. ▪ Follow the medial scapular border using the across and down pattern. ▪ Under the scapulas, stay in the midscapular line, percussing downward until resonance fades. (Normally resonance will disappear at about the 10th or 12th rib)			
23.	Diaphragmic Excursion ▪ Ask patient to exhale and hold breath. Percuss down the scapula line until the sound changes from resonance to dullness. Mark that spot.			

	▪ Ask patient to inhale and hold breathe. Percuss down from the 1st mark from resonance to dullness. ▪ Measure the difference between the marks. Diaphragmic motion is normally 4 to 6cm.			

	Auscultation (Posterior)	Completed Correctly	Omitted	Performed Incorrectly
24.	Have patient fold arms across the front of chest.			
25.	Ask patient to breathe in deeply through mouth and exhale with mouth open.			
26.	Using the diaphragm, Auscultate across and down pattern.			
27.	Listen to at least **6 key locations** (3 left and 3 right) beginning with the apices, and then follow the medial scapular borders.			

	Additional Techniques	Completed Correctly	Omitted	Performed Incorrectly
28.	**Wheezing:** Can be accentuated by a forced expiration.			
29.	**Rales:** May disappear after a few deep breaths and /or a cough.			
30.	**Whispered pectoriloquy:** Have patient whisper "one, two, three" while listening over the suspected lung field.			
31.	**Bronchophony:** Have patient speak, noting a change in intensity or clarity of the spoken voice over the suspected lung field. (blue moon, 99)			
32.	**Egophony:** Have patient vocalize the vowel "EEEE". It will be heard as the vowel A if the lung tissue is consolidated or compressed.			

PRACTICE WORKSHOP: VITAL SIGN EXAMINATION

	Introduction
1.	Student introduced self
2.	Student washed hands
3.	Student explained examination to the patient

	Assessment of Temperature
4.	Range (± 0.5 degrees) Manual thermometer or electronic thermometer reset and sheathed properly
	Thermometer inserted under frenulum
	Reading taken within 3-5 minutes Acceptable Temperature (Standard) *Range_____ °F to _____ °F

	Assessment of Pulse
5.	Range (± 20 bpm)
	Right arm recorded Left arm recorded
	*Range ____ bpm to ____ bpm

	Assessment of Respiration
6.	Student correctly assessed respiration without chest or shoulder contact. (okay to take pulse while measuring respiration) INCORRECT: Student tells patient s/he is checking respiration or touches shoulder or chest

	Assessment of Blood Pressure (Both arms)
7.	Made sure legs were uncrossed
8.	Palpated brachial artery
9.	Placed cuff in proper position
10.	Palpated radial artery

	Assessment of Blood Pressure	**Completed (+1)**	**Not Completed (-1)**	**Performed Incorrectly (-1)**
11.	Made sure legs were uncrossed			
12.	Palpated brachial artery			
13.	Placed cuff in proper position			
14.	Palpated radial artery			
15.	Assessed POP (inflated cuff until pulse diminished)			
16.	Deflated cuff completely and waited approximately 15 seconds			
17.	Inflated cuff again 20-30 mmHg above POP			

		Correct (+1)	**Not Correct (-1)**	**Student Response (mmHg)**
18.	**POP Range (± 10 mm Hg)** Acceptable **POP** (Standard) *Range ___mmHg to ___mmHg			
19.	**BP Range (± 5 mmHg)** Acceptable Blood Pressure (Standard) *Range___/___mmHg to ____/____mmHg			

INDEX:

Examinations and Assessments in Alphabetical Order

A

B

C

D

E

F

G

H

J

K

L

V

W

REFERENCES

Mangione S, Nieman LZ. Cardiac auscultatory skills of internal medicine and family practice trainees: A comparison of diagnostic proficiency. JAMA 1997; 278: 717-22.

Mangione S, Nieman LZ, Gracely E, Kaye D. The teaching and practice of cardiac auscultation during internal medicine and cardiology training: nationwide survey. Ann Intern Med 1993; 119: 47-54.

Nardone, Lucan LM, Palac DM. Physical examination: A revered skill under scrutiny. Southern Medical Journal 1988; 81: 770-73.

Sackett DL, Rennie D. The science of the art of the clinical examination. JAMA 1992; 267: 2650-52.

Sapira JD. Why perform a routine history and physical examination? Southern Medical Journal 1989; 82: 364-65.

Wiener S, Nathanson M. Physical examination: Frequently observed errors. JAMA 1976; 2: 852-55

Avorn J, Everitt DE, Baker MW. The neglected medical history and therapeutic choices for abdominal pain: A nationwide study of 799 physicians and nurses. Arch Intern Med 1991; 151: 694-98.

Bickley LS. Bates' Guide to Physical Exam and History Taking. 7th edition, Philadelphia; Lippincott 1999: 1-42.

Bingham J. On Being a Patient: A Complaint Against "Complaints." Ann Intern Med. 2003; 138: 73-74.
Hampton JR, Harrison, MJF, Mitchell JRA, Prichard JF, Sey-

mour C. Relative contributions of history-taking, physical examination, and laboratory investigation to diagnosis and management of medical outpatients. British Medical Journal 1975; 2: 486-89.

Oboler SK, LaForce M. The periodic physical examination in asymptomatic adults. Ann Intern Med 1989; 110: 214-26.

Peterson MC, Holbrook JH, Von Hales D, Smith NL, Staker LV. West J Med 1992; 156: 163-65.

Rich EC, Crowson TW, Harris IB. The diagnostic value of the medical history: Perceptions of internal medicine physicians. Arch Intern Med 1987; 147: 1957-60.

Sandler G. The importance of the history in the medical clinic and the cost of unnecessary tests. American Heart Journal 1980; 100: 928-31.

Sapira JD. The Art and Science of Bedside Diagnosis. 1st edition, Baltimore; Williams and Wilkins 1990: 1-46

Anand SS, et al. Does this patient have deep vein thrombosis? JAMA 1998; 279 (14): 1094-9.

Anderson MR, et al. Evaluation of vaginal complaints. JAMA 2004; 291 (11): 1368-79.

Bastian L, et al. Is this patient peri-menopausal? JAMA 2003; 289 (7): 895-902.

Bent S, et al. Does this woman have an acute uncomplicated urinary tract infection? JAMA 2002; 287 (20): 2701-10.

Bickley L. Bates' Guide to Physical Examination. 7th edition, Philadelphia; Lippincott Williams and Wilkins 1999: Review of Systems, 8-11.

Bradford J, et al. Blurred vision. NEJM 2000; 343 (8): 556-62.

Chunilal SD, et al. Does this patient have pulmonary embolism? JAMA 2003; 290 (21): 2849-58.

Cuker A, et al. A bloody mystery. NEJM 2009; 361 (19): 1887-94.

Degowin R, et al. Degowin's Diagnostic Examination. 7th edition. McGraw Hill 2000: Review of Systems, 29-31.

Detsky AS, et al. The rational clinical examination: Is this patient malnourished? JAMA 1994; 271 (1): 54-8.

Detsky ME, et al. Does this patient with headache have a migraine or need neuroimaging? JAMA 2006; 296 (10): 1274-83.

Deyo R, et al. Low back pain. NEJM 2001; 344 (5): 363-70.

Froehling DA, et al. The rational clinical examination: Does this dizzy patient have a serious form of vertigo? JAMA 1994; 271 (5): 385-8.

Goadsby P, et al. Migraine - Current understanding and treatment. NEJM 2002; 346 (4): 257-70.

Green P et al. Celiac disease. NEJM 2007; 357 (17): 1731-43.

Gross G. Review of Systems. Maine Medical Center, Dept of Internal Medicine. Nov 1989.

Hoffbrand BI. Away with the system review: a plea for parsimony. BMG 1989; 298: 817-9.

Holroyd-Leduc JM, et al. What type of urinary incontinence does this woman have? JAMA 2008; 299 (12): 1366-56.

Jacobs D. A 52 year-old suicidal man. JAMA 2000; 283: 2693-99.

Jager R, et al. Age related macular degeneration. NEJM 2008; 358(24): 2606-17.

Khan NA, et al. Does the clinical examination predict lower extremity peripheral arterial disease? JAMA 2006; 295 (5): 536-46.

Klompas M. Does this patient have an acute thoracic aortic dissection? JAMA 2002; 287 (17): 2262-72.

Margaretten ME, et al. Does this adult patient have septic arthritis? JAMA 2007; 297 (13): 1478-88.

Metlay J, et al. Does this patient have community-acquired pneumonia? Diagnosing pneumonia by history and physical examination. JAMA 1997; 278 (17): 1440-5.

Mitchell TL, et al. Yield of the screening review of systems: a study on a general medical service. JGIM 1992; 7 (4): 393-7

Panju A, et al. The rational clinical examination. Is this patient having a myocardial infarction? JAMA 1998; 280 (14); 1256-63.

Rao G, et al. Does this patient have Parkinson disease? JAMA 2003; 289 (3); 347-53.

Schwenk T. Screening for depression in primary Care. JAMA 2000; 284 (11): 1379-80.

Schwenk T. Screening for depression in primary care: a disease in search of a test; JGIM 1996; 11: 437-9.

Sharpe M, wt al. ABC of psychological medicine. BMJ 2002; 325: 480-3.

Swartz MH. Swartz Textbook of Physical Diagnosis: History and Examination. 4th edition, WB Saunders 2002: Review of Systems, 28-30.

Silen W. Cope's early diagnosis of the acute abdomen. 17th edition. Oxford University Press 1987.

Trowbridge RL, et al. Does this patient have acute cholecystitis? JAMA 2003; 289 (1): 80-6.

Wagner J. Does this patient have appendicitis? JAMA 1996; 276 (19): 1589-94.

Wang CS, et al. Does this dyspneic patient in the emergency department have congestive heart failure? JAMA 2005; 294 (15) 1944-56.

Wells PS, et al. Does this patient have deep ein thrombosis? JAMA 2006; 295 (2): 199-207.

Whited JD, et al. The rational clinical examination: Does this patient have a mole or a melanoma? JAMA 1998; 279 (9): 696-701.

Williams J. Is this patient clinically depressed? JAMA 2002; 287 (9):1160-70.

Williams JW, et al. Does this patient have sinusitis? Diagnosing acute sinusitis by history and physical examination. JAMA 1993; 270 (10): 1242-6.

VITAL SIGNS

American Heat Association. Recommendations for human blood pressure determination by sphygmomanometers. American Heart Association Publication 1980.

Benowitz NL, Kuyt F, Jacob P. Influence of nicotine on cardiovascular and hormonal effects of cigarette smoking. Clin Pharmacol Ther 1984; 36: 74-81.

Bickley LS. Bates' Guide to Physical Exam and History Taking. 7th edition, Philadelphia; Lippincott 1999: 292-99.

Caird FI, Andrew GR, Kennedy RD. Effect of posture on blood pressure in the elderly. British Heart Journal 1973; 35: 527-30.

Corley DA, Stefan AM, Wolf M, Cook F, Lee TH. Early indicators of prognosis in upper gastrointestinal hemorrhage. Am J Gastroenterology 1998; 93: 336-340.

Crenner CW. Introduction of the blood pressure cuff into U.S. medical practice: Technology and skilled practice. Ann Intern Med 1998; 128: 488-93.

Frohlich ED, Grim C, Labarthe DR, Maxwell MH, Perloff D, Weidman WH. Recommendations for human blood pressure determination by sphygmomanometers: Report of a special task force appointed by the steering committee, American Heart Association. Hypertension 1988; 11: 210a-221a.

Joint national committee on prevention, detection, and treatment of high blood pressure and the national high blood pressure education program coordinating committee. The sixth report of the joint national committee on prevention, detection, evaluation and treatment of high blood pressure. Arch Intern Med 1997; 157: 2413-2443.

Kollef MH, O'Brien JD, Zuckerman GR, Shannon W. BLEED: A classification tool to predict outcomes in patients with acute upper and lower gastrointestinal hemorrhage. Crit Care Med 1997; 25: 1125-32.

Koziol-McLain J, Lowenstein SR, Fuller B. Orthostatic vital signs in emergency department patients. Ann Emerg Med 1991; 20: 606-10.

Londe S, Klitzner TS. Auscultatory blood pressure measurement - Effect of pressure on the head of the stethoscope. West J Med 1984; 141: 193-95.

Maxwell MH, Waks AU, Schroth PC, Karam M, Dornfeld LP. Error in blood-pressure measurement due to incorrect cuff size in obese patients. Lancet July 3, 1982; 33-35.

McGee S, Abernethy WB, Simerl DL. Is this patient hypovolemic? JAMA 1999; 281: 1022-29.

McGrady A, Higgins JT. Effect of repeated measurements of blood pressure on blood pressure in essential hypertension: Role of anxiety. J of Behavioral Medicine 1990; 13: 93-101.

O'Brien ET, O'Malley. ABC of blood pressure measurement: The patient. British Medical Journal October 13, 1979: 920-21.

O'Brien ET, O'Malley. ABC of blood pressure measurement: The sphygmomanometer. British Medical Journal October 6, 1979: 851-53.

O'Brien ET, O'Malley. ABC of blood pressure measurement: Technique. British Medical Journal October 20, 1979: 982-84.

Reeves RA. Does this patient have hypertension? How to measure blood pressure. JAMA 1995; 273: 1211-18.

Russell AE, Wing LMH, Smith SA, Aylward PE, McRitchie RJ, Hassam RM, West MJ, Chalmers JP. Optimal size of cuff bladder for indirect measurement of arterial pressure in adults. J of Hypertension 1989; 7: 607-613.

Sapira JD. The Art and Science of Bedside Diagnosis. 1st edition, Baltimore; Williams and Wilkins 1990: 139-53; 85-104.

Scherwitz LW, Evans LA, Hennrikus DJ, Vallbona C. Procedures and discrepancies of blood pressure measurements in two community health centers. Medical Care 1982; 20: 727-38.

Silverberg DS, Shemesh E, Iaina A. The unsupported arm: A cause of falsely raised blood pressure readings. British Medical Journal November 19, 1977; 1331.

Smith TDW, Clayton D. Individual variation between general practitioners in labeling of hypertension. British Medical Journal 1990; 300: 74-75.

Steinfeld L, Alexander H, Cohen ML. Updating sphygmomanometry. Am J of Cardiol 1974; 33: 107-10.

Viol GW, Goebel M, Lorenz GJ, Ing TS. Seating as a variable in clinical blood pressure measurement. American Heart Journal 1979; 98: 813-14.

Waaler HT. Specificity and sensitivity of blood pressure measurements. J of Epidemiology and Comm Health 1980; 34: 53-58.

Ward C, Kenny RA. Reproducibility of orthostatic hypotension in symptomatic elderly. Am J of Med 1996; 100: 418-22.

Webb CH. The measurement of blood pressure and its interpretation. Primary Care 1980; 7: 637-51.

Taler S. Initial treatment of hypertension. NEJM 2018; 378:636-644.

ACC/AHA Task force. 2017 ACC/AHA/AAPA/ABC/ACPM/AGS/APhA/ASH/ASPC/NMA/PCNA Guideline for the Prevention, Detection, Evaluation, and Management of High Blood Pressure in Adults. Hypertension 2017. 1-283.

Carey R, et al. Prevention, Detection, Evaluation, and Management of High Blood Pressure in Adults: Synopsis of the 2017 American College of Cardiology/American Heart Association Hypertension Guideline. Annals Int Med 2018; 168: 351-8.

THE EYE EXAM

Bickley LS. Bates' Guide to Physical Exam and History Taking. 7th edition, Philadelphia; Lippincott 1999: 163-70, 184-95, 211-27.

Leibowitz HM. The red eye. NEJM 2000; 343: 345-51.

McGee S. Evidence based physical diagnosis, 2nd ed. Chapter 19: The pupils. Saunders 2007: 209-241.

Sapira JD. The Art and Science of Bedside Diagnosis. 1st edition, Baltimore; Williams and Wilkins 1990: 139-53; 155-205.

Shingleton BJ, O'Donoghue. Blurred vision. NEJM 2000; 343: 556-62.

Shingleton BJ. Eye injuries. NEJM 1991;325: 408-13.

Vaughan D, Asbury T, Riordan-Eva P. General ophthalmology. 15th edition, Stamford; Appleton and Lange 1999.

Wu G. Ophthalmology for primary care. 1st edition, Philadelphia; W.B. Saunders Company 1997.

HEAD AND NECK EXAM

Bagai A, Thavendiranathan P, Detsky A. Does This Patient Have Hearing Impairment? JAMA 2006; 295: 416 - 428.

Bickley LS. Bates' Guide to Physical Exam and History Taking. 7th edition, Philadelphia; Lippincott 1999: 163-244.

Brander A, Viikinkoski P, Tuuhea J, Voutilainene L, Kivisaari L. Clinical versus ultrasound examination of the thyroid gland in common clinical practice. J Clin Ultrasound 1992; 20: 37-42.

Ferrer R. Lymphadenopathy: Differential diagnosis and evaluation. American Family Physician 1998; 58: 1313-20.

Habermann TM, Steensma DP. Lymphadenopathy. Mayo Clin Proc 2000; 75: 723-32.

Jarlov AE, Hegedus L, Gjorup T, Hansen JM. Observer variation in the clinical assessment of the thyroid gland. Journal of Internal Medicine 1991; 229: 159-61.

Kennedy D. A 48-year old man with recurrent sinusitis. JAMA 2000; 283: 2143-2150.

Linet OI, Metzler C. Incidence of palpable cervical nodes in adults. Postgraduate Medicine 1977; 62: 210-13.

Pangalis GA, Vassilakopoulos TP, Boussiotis A, Fessas P. Clinical approach to lymphadenopathy. Seminars in Oncology 1993; 20: 570-82.

Sapira JD. The Art and Science of Bedside Diagnosis. 1st edition, Baltimore; Williams and Wilkins 1990: 139-53; 207-237.

Siminoski K. Does this patient have a goiter? JAMA 1995; 273: 813-17.

Slap GB, Brooks JSJ, Schwartz S. When to perform biopsies of enlarged peripheral lymph nodes in young patients. JAMA 1984; 252: 1321-26.

Williams JW, Simel DL. Does this patient have sinusitis? Diagnosing acute sinusitis by history and physical examination. JAMA 1993; 279: 1242-46.

Acres JC, Kryger MH. Clinical significance of pulmonary function tests: Upper airway obstruction. Chest 1981; 80: 207-11.

Andrews JL, Badger TL. Lung sounds through the ages: From Hippocreates to Laennec to Osler. JAMA 1979; 241: 2625-30.

Badgett RG, Tanaka DJ, Hunt DK, Jelley MJ, Feinberg LE, Steiner JF, Petty TL. Can moderate chronic obstructive pulmonary disease be diagnosed by historical and physical findings alone? Am J of Med 1993; 94: 188-96.

Bickley LS. Bates' Guide to Physical Exam and History Taking. 7th edition, Philadelphia; Lippincott, 1999: 245-75.

Forgacs P. The functional basis of pulmonary sounds. Chest 1978; 73: 399-405.

Forgacs P. Lung sounds. Brit J Dis Chest 1969; 63: 1-12.

Heckerling PS, Tape TG, Wigton RS, Hissong KK, Leikin JB, Ornato JP, Cameron JL, Racht EM. Clinical prediction rule for pulmonary infiltrates. Ann Intern Med 1990; 113: 664-70.

Holleman DR, Simel DL. Does the clinical examination predict airflow limitation? JAMA 1995; 273: 313-19.

King DK, Thompson T, Johnson DC. Wheezing on maximal forced exhalation in the diagnosis of atypical asthma: Lack of sensitivity and specificity. Ann Intern Med 1989; 110: 451-55.

Loudon R, Murphy RLH. Lung sounds. Am Rev Respir Dis 1984; 130: 663-73.

Mannino DM, Etzel RA, Flanders D. Do the medical history and physical examination predict low lung function? Arch Intern Med 1993; 153: 1892-97.

Metlay JP, Kapoor WN, Fine MJ. Does this patient have community-acquired pneumonia? JAMA 1997; 278: 1440-45.

Osmer JC, Cole BK. The stethoscope and roentgenogram in acute pneumonia. Southern Med J 1966; 59: 75-77.

Sapira JD. The Art and Science of Bedside Diagnosis. 1st edition, Baltimore; Williams and Wilkins 1990: 245-81.

Schapira JM, Schapira MM, Funahashi A, McAuliffe TL, Varkey B. The value of the forced expiratory time in the physical diagnosis of obstructive airways disease. JAMA 1993; 270: 731-36.

Singal BM, Hedges JR, Radack KL. Decision rules and clinical prediction of pneumonia: Evaluation of low-yield criteria. Ann Emerg Med 1989; 18: 13-20.

Spiter MA, Cook DG, Clarke SW. Reliability of eliciting physical signs in examination of the chest. Lancet April 16, 1988: 873 -75.

Stubbing DG Mathur PN, Roberts RS, Campbell EJM. Some physical signs in patients with chronic airflow obstruction. Am Rev Respir Dis 1982; 125: 549-52.

Thacker RE, Kraman SS. The prevalence of auscultatory crackles in subjects without lung disease. Chest 1982; 6: 672-74.

Weinberger S. Principles of Pulmonary Medicine. 1st edition, Philadelphia; W.B. Saunders Company 1986.

West JB. Respiratory Physiology. 4th edition, Baltimore; Williams and Wilkins 1990.

West JB. Pulmonary Pathophysiology. 4th edition, Baltimore; Williams and Wilkins 1992.

Wilkins RL, Dexter JR, Murphy RLH, DelBono EA. Lung sound nomenclature survey. Chest 1990; 98: 886-89

Bladgett RG, Lucey CR, Mulrow CD. Can the clinical examination diagnose left-sided heart failure in adults? JAMA 1997; 277: 1712-19.

Bethell HJN, Nixon PG. Cardiovascular Exam in supine and left lateral positions. British Heart Journal 1973: 35: 902-7.

Bickley LS. Bates' Guide to Physical Exam and History Taking. 7th edtion, Philadelphia; Lippincott, 1999: 277-332.

Braunwald E (editor). Heart Disease: A Textbook of Cardiovascular Medicine. 5th edition, Philadelphia; W.B. Saunders Co.: 15 -52.

Carabello BA, Crawford FA. Valvular heart disease. NEJM 1997; 337: 32-41.

Chambers BR, Norris JW. Outcome in patients with asymptomatic neck bruits. NEJM 1986; 315: 860-65.

Choudhyr NK, Echells EE. Does this patient have aortic regurgitation? JAMA 1999; 281: 2231-38.

Chun PKD, Dunn BE. Clinical clue of severe aortic stenosis: Simultaneous palpation of the carotid and apical impulses. Arch Inern Med 1982; 142: 2284-88.

Conn DC, Cole JS. The cardiac apex impulse: Clinical and angiographic correlation. Ann Intern Med 1971; 75: 185-91.

Constant J. Bedside Cardiology. 4th edition, Boston; Little, Brown and Co.; 1993.

Cook DJ, Simel DL. Does this patient have abnormal central venous pressure? JAMA 1996; 275: 630-34.

Cooperman M, Martin EW, Evans WE. Significance of asymptomatic carotid bruits. Arch Surg 1978; 113: 1339-40.

Curtiss EI, Matthews RG, Shaver JA. Mechanism of normal splitting of the second heart sound. Circulation 1975; 51: 157-64.

Davison R, Cannon R. Estimation of central venous pressure by examination of jugular veins. American Heart Journal 1974; 87: 279-82.

Ducas J, Magder S, McGregor M. Validity of the hepatojugular reflux as a clinical test of congestive heart failure. American Journal of Cardiology 1983; 52: 1299-1303.

Eagle KA, Quertermous T, Singer DE, Mulley AG, Reder VA, Boucher C, Strauss HW, Thibault GE. Left ventricular ejection fraction: Physician estimates compared with gated blood pool scan measurements. Arch Intern Med 1988; 148: 882-85.

Eilern SD, Crawford MH, O'Rourke RA. Accuracy of precordial palpation for detecting increased left ventricular volume. Ann Intern Med 1983; 99: 628-30.

Eisenberg PR, Jaffe AS, Schuster DP. Clinical evaluation compared to pulmonary artery catheterization in the hemodynamic assessment of critically ill patients. Critical Care Medicine 1984; 12: 549-53.

Etchells E, Bell C, Robb K. Does this patient have an abnormal systolic murmur? JAMA 1997; 277: 564-71.

Executive committee for the asymtpomatic carotid atherosclerosis study. Endarterectomry for asymptomatic carotid artery stenosis. JAMA 1995; 273: 1421-28.

Ghail JK, Kadakia S, Cooper R, Liao Y. Bedside diagnosis of preserved versus impaired left ventricular systolic function in heart failure. American Journal of Cardiology 1991; 67: 1002-06.

Harvey WP. Cardiac Pearls. Disease-a-Month 1994; Mosby: 43-112.

Heyman A, Wilkinson WE, Heyden S, Helms MJ, Bartel AG,

Karp HR, Tyroloer HA, Hames CG. Risk of stroke in asymptomatic persons with cervical arterial bruits: A population study in Evans County, Georgia. NEJM 1980; 302: 838-41.

Hurst JW, Hopkins LC, Smith RB. Noises in the neck. NEJM 1980; 302: 362-62.

Lembro NJ, DellÍtalia LJ, Crawford MH, O'Rourke RA. Bedside diagnosis of systolic murmurs. NEJM 1988; 318: 1572-78.

Maisel A, Atwood E, Goldberger AL. Hepatojugular reflux: Useful in the bedside diagnosis of tricuspid regurgitation. Ann Int Med 1984; 101: 781-81.

Mattelman SJ, Hakki A, Iskandrian AS, Segal BL, Kane SA. Reliability of beside evaluation in determining left ventricular function: Correlation with left ventricular ejection fraction determined by radionuclide ventriculography. J Am Coll Cardiol 1983; 1 (2): 417-20.

Munro NC, McIntoh S, Lawson J, Morley C, Sutton R, Kenny RA. Incidence of complications after carotid sinus massage in older patients with syncope. J American Geriatric Soc 1994; 42: 1248-51.

Meyers DG, Sagar KB, Ingram RF, Paulsen WJ, Romhilt DW. Diagnosis of aortic insufficiency: Comparison of auscultation and m-mode echocardiography to angiography. Southern Medical Journal 1982; 75: 1192-94.

Nellen M, Gotsman MS, Vogelpoel L, Beck W, Schrire V. Effects of prompt squatting on the systolic murmur in idiopathic hypertrophic obstructive cardiomyopathy. British Medical Journal 1967; 3: 140-43.

North American symtpomatic carotid endarterectomy trial collaborators. Beneficial effect of carotid endarterecomy in symptomatic patients with high-grade stenosis. NEJM 1991; 325: 445-53.

O'Rourke MF. The arterial pulse in health and disease. American Heart Journal 1971; 82: 687-702.

Rahko PS. Prevalence of regurgitant murmurs in patients with valvular regurgitation detected by doppler echocardiography. Ann Intern Med 1989; 111: 466-72.

Rosenblum R, Delman AJ. Valsalva's maneuver and the systolic murmur of hypertrophic subaortic stenosis: A bediside diagnostic test. American Journal of Cardiology 1965; 15:868-70.

Roederer GO, Langlois YE, Jager KA, Primozich BS, Beach KW, Phillips DJ, Strandness DE. The natural history of carotid arterial disease in asymptomatic patients with cervical bruits. Stroke 1984; 15: 605-13.

Roldan C, Shively BK, Crawford MH. Value of the cardiovascular physical examination for detecting valvular heart disease in asymptomatic subjects. American Journal of Cardiology 1996: 77: 1327-31.

Sapira JD. The Art and Science of Bedside Diagnosis. 1st edition, Baltimore; Williams and Wilkins 1990: 283-370.

Sauve JS, Laupacis A, Ostbye T, Feagan B, Sacett DL. Does this patient have a clinically important carotid bruit? JAMA 1993; 270: 2843-45.

Schlant RC (editor). The Heart, Arteries and Veins. 8th edition, New York; McGraw-Hill, Inc.; 229-51.

Stoelting RK. Evaluation of right atrial pressure. Anesthesiology 1973; 38: 291-94.

Van Ruiswyk J, Noble H, Sigmann. The natural history of carotid bruits in elderly persons. Ann Intern Med 1990; 112: 340-43.

Vongpatanasin W, Hillis LD, Lange A. Prosthetic heart valves. NEJM 1996; 335: 407-16.

Wang C, Fitzgerald J, Schulzer M, Mak E, Ayas N. Does This Dyspneic Patient in the Emergency Department Have Congestive Heart Failure? JAMA 2005; 294: 1944 - 1956.

Westman EC, Matchar DB, Samsa GP, Mulrow CD, Waugh RA, Feussner JF. Accuracy and reliability of apical s3 gallop detection. Journal of General Internal Medicine 1995; 455-57.

Wolf PA, Kannel WB, Sorlie P, McNamara P. Asymptomatic carotid bruit and risk of stroke: The Framingham study. JAMA 1981; 245: 1442-45.

Arnell TD, de Virgilio C, Donayre C, Grant E, Baker JD, White R. Abdominal aortic aneurysm screening in elderly males with atherosclerosis: The value of physical exam. The American Surgeon 1996; 62: 861-64.

Barkun AN, Camus M, Green L, Meagher T, Coupal L, de Stempel , Grover S. The bedside assessment of splenic enlargement. The American Journal of Medicine 1991; 91: 512-18.

Bickley LS. Bates' Guide to Physical Exam and History Taking. 7th edition, Philadelphia; Lippincott, 1999: 355-86.

Castell C. How big is the normal liver, indeed! Arch Intern Med 1979; 139: 968-9.

Castell DO. The spleen percussion sign: A useful diagnostic technique. Ann Intern Med 1967; 67: 1265-67.

Castell DO, O'Brien KD, Muench H, Chalmers TC. Estimation of liver size by percussion in normal individuals. Ann Intern Med 1969; 70: 1183-89.

Chervu A, Clagett P, Valentine J, Myers SI, Rossi PJ. Role of physical examination in detection of abdominal aortic aneurysms. Surgery 1995; 117: 454-57.

Cumings S, Papadakis M, Melnick J, Gooding GAW, Tierney LM. The predictive value of physical examinations for ascites. West J Med 1985; 142: 633-36.

Eippe DF, Gifford RW, Stewart BH, Alfidi RJ, McCormack LJ, Vidt DG. Abdominal bruits in renovascular hypertension. Am J of Cardioll 1976; 37: 48-52.

Ebaugh FG, McIntyre OR. Palpable spleens: Ten-year follow-up. Ann Intern Med 1979; 90: 130-31.

Fink HA, Lederle FA, Roth CS, Bowles C, Nelson DB, Haas MA. The accuracy of physical examination to detect abdominal aortic aneurysm. Arch Intern Med 2000; 160: 833-36.

Fuller GN, Hargreaves MR, King DM. Scratch test in clinical examination of liver. Lancet January 23, 1988; 181.

Goldberg BB, Clearfield HR, Goodman GA, Morales JO. Ultrasonic determination of ascites. Arch Intern Med 1973; 131: 217-20.

Grover SA, Barkun AN, Sackett DL. Does this patient have splenomegaly? JAMA 1993; 270: 2218-21.

Guarino JR. Auscultatory percussion to detect ascites. NEJM 1986; 315: 1555-56.

Julius S, Stewart BH. Diagnostic significance of abdominal murmurs. NEJM 1967; 276: 1175-78.

Kiev J, Eckhardt A, Kerstein MD. Reliability and accuracy of physical examination in detection of abdominal aortic aneurysms. Vascular Surgery 1997; 31: 143-46.

Lederle FA, Simel DL. Does this patient have abdominal aortic aneurysm? JAMA 1999; 281: 77-82.

Lederle FA, Walker JM, Reinke DB. Selective screening for abdominal aortic aneurysms with physical examination and ultrasound. Arch Intern Med 1988; 148: 1753-56.

McClouglin MJ, Colapinto RF, Hobbs BB. Abdominal bruits: Clinical and angiographic correlation. JAMA 1975; 232: 1238-42.

Naylor CD. Physical examination of the liver. JAMA 1994; 271: 1859-65.

Rivin AU. Abdominal vascular sounds. JAMA 1972; 221: 688-90.

Simon N, Franklin SS, Bleifer KH, Maxwell MH. Clinical characteristics of renovascular hypertension. JAMA 1972; 220: 1209 -18.

Sapira JD. The Art and Science of Bedside Diagnosis. 1st edition, Baltimore; Williams and Wilkins 1990: 371-90.

Sapira JD, Williamson DL. How big is the normal liver? Arch Intern Med 1979; 139: 971-73.

Silen W. Cope's early diagnosis of the acute abdomen. 17th edition, New York; Oxford Press 1987.

Skrainka B, Stahlhut J, Fulbeck CL, Knight F, Holmes RA, Butt JH. Measuring liver span. J Clin Gastroenterol 1986; 8: 267-70.

Sullivan S, Krasner N, Williams R. The clinical estimation of liver size: A comparison of techniques and an analysis of the source of error. British Medical Journal 1976; 2: 1042-43.

Turnbull JM. Is listening for abdominal bruits useful in the evaluation of hypertension? JAMA 1995; 274: 1299-1301.

Wagner JM, McKinney P, Carpenter JL. Does this patient have appendicitis? JAMA 1996; 276: 1589-94.

Williams JW, Simel DL. Does this patient have ascites? JAMA 1992; 267: 2645-48.

Adams K. Lump detection in simulated human breasts. Perception and Psychophysicis 1976; 20: 163-7.

Baines C, Miller A, Bassett A. Physical examination. Its role as a single screening modality in the Canadian national breast screening study. Cancer 1989; 63: 1816-22.

Baines CJ, Miller AB. Mammography versus clinical examination of the breasts. J Natl Cancer Institute Monographs 1997; 22: 125-9.

Baines CJ. Physical examination of the breasts in screening for breast cancer. J Gerontol 1992; 47: 63-7.

Barnes C. Breast palpation technique: what is the finer pad? J Chronic Disease 1987; 40: 361-2.

Barton M, Harris R, Fletcher S. Does this patient have breast cancer?: The screening clinical breast examination: Should it be done? How? JAMA 1999; 282: 1270-80.

Bickley LS. Bates' Guide to Physical Exam and History Taking. 9th edition, Philadelphia; Lippincott 2007: 337-357 .

Bloom HS, Criswell E, Pennypacker H. . Major stimulus dimensions determining detection of simulated breast lesions. Perception and Psychophysiology 1982; 32: 251-60.

Campbell HS, Fletcher SW, Pilgrim CA, Morgan TM, Lin S. Improving physicians and nurses clinical breast examination: A randomized controlled trial. Am J Prev Med 1991; 7: 1-8.

Donegan W. Evaluation of a palpable breast mass. NEJM 1992; 327: 937-42.

Fletcher S, O'Malley M, Earp J, Morgan T, Lin S, Dengan D. How best to teach women breast self-examination: A randomized controlled trial. Ann Int Med 1990; 112: 772-9.

Gulay H, Bora S. Management of nipple discharge. J Am Coll Surg 1994; 178: 471-4.

Hall D, Goldstein M, Stein G. Progress in manual breast examination. Cancer 1977; 40: 364-70.

Hall D, Adams C, Stein G, Stephenson H, Goldstein M. Improved detection of human breast lesions following experimental training. Cancer 1980; 46: 408-14.

Kerlikowske K, Simth-Bindman R, Ljung B, Grady D. Evaluation of abnormal mammography results and palpable breast abnormalities. Ann Intern Med 2003; 139: 274-84.

Love S, Gelman R, Silen W. Sounding board. Fibrocystic "disease of the breast - a nondisease? NEJM 1982; 307: 1010-4.

Mahoney L, Csima A. Efficiency of palpation in clinical detection of breast cancer. Can Med Assoc J 1982; 127: 729-30.

McDermott M, Dolan N, Huang J, Reifler D, Rademaker A. Lump detection is enhanced in silicone breast models stimulating postmenopausal breast tissue. JGen Intern Med 1996; 11: 112-4.

Mushlin A. Diagnostic tests in breast cancer. Clinical strategies based on diagnostic possibilities. Ann Int Med 1985; 103: 79-85.

Pilgrim C, Lannon C, Harris R, Cogburn W, Fletcher S. Improving clinical breast examination training in a medical school: A randomized trial. J of Gen Int Med 1993; 8: 685-8.

Sanders K, Pilgrim C, Pennypacker H. Increased proficiency of search in breast self exam. Cancer 1986; 58: 2531-7.

Sapira JD. The Art and Science of Bedside Diagnosis. 1st edition, Baltimore; Williams and Wilkins 1990: 239-43.

Screening for breast cancer; Summary of recommendations. U.S. Preventative Services Task Force (USPSTF). 2002. http://www.ahrq.gov/clinic/uspstf/uspsbrca.htm

Stephenson HS, Adams CK, Hall DC, Pennypacker HS. Effects of certain training parameters on detection of simulated breast cancer. Journal of Behavioral Medicine 1979; 2: 239-50.

Winchester D. Physical examination of the breast. Cancer 1992; 69: 1947-9.

Barnhart K. Ectopic pregnancy. NEJM 2009; 361: 379-87

Basson R. Sexual desire and arousal disorders in women. NEJM 2006; 354:1497-150.

Bastian L, et al. Is this patient perimenopausal? JAMA. 2003; 289(7): 895-902.

Biggs W, et al. Diagnosis and Management of Adnexal Masses. Am Fam Phys 2016; 93(8): 676-681.

Bulun S. Uterine fibroids. NEJM 2013; 369:1344-1355.

Committee on Gyn Practice. Management of acute abnormal uterine bleeding in non-pregnant reproductive-aged women. Committee opinion 557, ACOG, April 2013.

Crochet J, et al. Does This Woman Have an Ectopic Pregnancy? JAMA. 2013; 309(16): 1722-1729.

Eckert L. Acute vulvovaginitis. NEJM 2006; 355: 1244-52.

Edelman A, et al. Pelvic Exam, NEJM Videos In Medicine Series. NEJM 2007; 356; e26. Accessed 7/2018.

Hoffman BL, et al. Chapter 33. Endometrial Cancer. In: Williams Gynecology, 2e. New York, NY: McGraw-Hill; 2012.

Hoffman BL, et al. Chapter 8. Abnormal Uterine Bleeding. In: Williams Gynecology, 2e. New York, NY: McGraw-Hill; 2012.

Hoffman BL, et al. Chapter 9. Pelvic Mass. In: Williams Gynecology, 2e. New York, NY: McGraw-Hill; 2012

Hopkins M, et al. BMJ Best Practices: Ovarian Torsion - Symptoms, diagnosis and treatment. https://bestpractice.bmj.com/topics/en-us/792. Accessed 7/2018.

Potter J, Carrion-Gomez Y. The Pelvic Exam Web Site and Videos. The Carl J Shapiro Institute for Education and Research at the Harvard Medical School and Beth Israel Deaconess Medical Center. https://research.bidmc.harvard.edu/vptutorials/midlife/tutorialShow.asp?setID=10710&1&openChapter=none Accessed 7/2018.

Surette A, et al, eds. CURRENT Diagnosis & Treatment: Obstetrics & Gynecology, 11e. Chapter 13. Early Pregnancy Risks. NY, NY: McGraw-Hill; 2013.

Sweet M, et al. Evaluation and management of abnormal uterine bleeding in premenopausal women. Am Fam Phys 2012; 85 (1): 35-43.

Wilson J. Vaginitis and cervicitis. Ann Intern Med. 2009;151 (5):ITC3-1.

Bickley LS. Bates' Guide to Physical Exam and History Taking. 7th edtion, Philadelphia; Lippincott, 1999: 387-403; 449-59.

Dixon JM, Elton RA, Rainey JB, Macleod DAD. Rectal examination in patients with pain in the right lower quadrant of the abdomen. British Medical Journal 1991; 302: 386-88.

Sapira JD. The Art and Science of Bedside Diagnosis. 1st edition, Baltimore; Williams and Wilkins 1990: 391-98, 411-14.

Wantz GE. A 65 year old man with an inguinal hernia. JAMA 1997; 277: 663-69.

Bickley LS. Bates' Guide to Physical Exam and History Taking. 7th edtion, Philadelphia; Lippincott, 1999: 461-68.

Dorrington KL. Skin turgor: Do we understand the clinical sign? Lancet January 31, 1981; 264-65.

Myers KA, Farquhar DRE. Does This Patient Have Clubbing? The Rational Clinical Examination. JAMA 2001; 286: 341-347.

Sapira JD. The Art and Science of Bedside Diagnosis. 1st edition, Baltimore; Williams and Wilkins 1990: 435-42.

Schriger DL, Baraff LJ. Capillary refill - Is it a useful predictor of hypovolemic states? Ann Emerg Med 1991; 20: 601-605.

Schriger DL, Baraff L. Defining normal capillary refill: Variation with age, sex and temperature. Ann Emerg Med 1988; 17: 932-35.

Shneerson JM. Digital clubbing and hypertrophic osteoarthropathy: The underlying mechanisms. Br J Dis Chest 1981; 75: 113-25.

The Book of Physical Diagnosis by Mark H. Swartz, Seventh Edition

Anand SS, Wells PS, Hunt D, Brill-Edwards P, Cook D, Ginsberg JS. Does this patient have deep vein thrombosis? JAMA 1998; 279: 1094-99.

Barnes RW, Wu KK, Hoak JC. Fallibility of the clinical diagnosis of venous thrombosis. JAMA 1975; 234: 605-07.

Bickley LS. Bates' Guide to Physical Exam and History Taking. 7th Edtion, Philadelphia; Lippincott, 1999: 461-82.

Blankfield RP, Findelhor RS, Alexander JJ, Flocke SA, Maiocco J, Goodwin M, Zyzanski SJ. Etiology and diagnosis of bilateral leg edema in primary care. American Journal of Medicine 1998; 105: 192-97.

Caputo GM, Cavanagh PR, Ulbrecht JS, Gibbons GW, Karchmer AW. Assessment and management of foot disease in patients with diabetes. NEJM 1994; 331: 854-60.

Cymet TC, Weisman DS. Lower leg ulcers. Hospital Physician July, 1997; 30-41.

Haeger K. Problems of acute deep venous thrombosis: The interpretation of signs and symptoms. Angiology 1969; 20: 219-223.

Hirsh J, Hull RD, Raskob GE. Clinical features and diagnosis of venous thrombosis. J Am Coll Cardiol 1986; 8: 114B-127B.

Loscalzo J (editor). Vascular Medicine: A textbook of vascular biology and diseases. 1st edition, Boston; Little, Brown and Compay 1992: 401-18.

Merli GJ, Spandorfer J. The outpatient with unilateral leg swelling. Medical clinics of North America 1995; 79: 435-47.

Nelzen O, Bergqvist D, Lindhagen A. Venous and non-venous ulcers: Clinical history and appearance in a population study. British Journal of Surgery 1995; 81: 182-87.

Sapira JD. The Art and Science of Bedside Diagnosis. 1st edition, Baltimore; Williams and Wilkins 1990: 442-49.

Sumpio BE. Foot ulcers. NEJM 2000; 343: 787-92.

Vaughan BF. CT of swollen legs. Clinical Radiology 1990; 41: 24-30.

Wells PS, Hirsh J, Andeson DR, Lensing AWA, Foster G, Kearon C, Weitz J, D'Ovidio, Cogo A, Prandoni P, Girolami A, Ginsberg JS. Accuracy of clinical assessment of deep-vein thrombosis. Lancet 1995; 345: 1326-30.

Bickley LS. Bates' Guide to Physical Exam and History Taking. 7th edtion, Philadelphia; Lippincott, 1999: 107-27.

Froehlich TE, Robison JT, Inouye SK. Screening for dementia in the outpatient setting: The time and change test. J American Geriatrics Soc 1998; 46: 1506-11.

Hirschfeld RMA, Russell JM. Assessment and treatment of suicidal patients. NEJM 1997; 337: 910-15.

Lipowski, ZJ. Delirium (acute confusional states). JAMA 1987; 258: 1789-92.

Lipowski ZJ. Delirium in the elderly patient. NEJM 1989; 320: 578-82.

Small SM. Outline for psychiatric examination: 6-21.

Sapira JD. The Art and Science of Bedside Diagnosis. 1st edition, Baltimore; Williams and Wilkins 1990: 516-22.

Adkins S, Figler R. Hip pain in athletes. American Family Physician 2000; 61: 2109-20.

Anto C, Aradhya P. Clinical diagnosis of peripheral nerve compression in the upper extremity. Orthopedic Clinics of North America 1996; 27: 227-236.

Baker D, Schumacher H. Acute monoarthritis. NEJM 1993; 329: 1013-20.

Bernstein J, Ivins D. Impingement syndrome: differential diagnosis and treatment strategies. Hospital Medicine 1999 (Oct): 24 -29.

Bickley LS. Bates' Guide to Physical Exam and History Taking. 7th edition, Philadelphia; Lippincott 1999: 483-5532.

Boyd R. Evaluation of back pain. Primary Care Medicine (Goroll A, Editor), 3rd Edition, Philadelphia; Lippincott 1995: 742-51.

Burkhart S. A 26-year-old woman with shoulder pain. JAMA 2000; 284: 1559-67.

Campbell CS. Gamekeeper's Thumb. The Journal of Bone and Joint Surgery1955; 37B: 148-49.

Canale TS. Campbell's Operative Orthopaedics 10th Ed., Philadelphia; Mosby: 2180-2211.

Cardone D, Tallia A. Diagnostic and therapeutic injection of the elbow region. American Family Physician 2002; 66: 2097-100.
Carragee E. Persistent low back pain. NEJM 2005; 352: 1891-98.

Chapman MW. Chapman's Orthopaedic Surgery 3rd Ed., Philadelphia; Lippincott: 2247-2265.

Chumbley E, O'Connor F, Nirschl R. Evaluation of overuse elbow injuries. American Family Physician 2000; 61: 691-702.

Colman W, Strauch R. Physical examination of the elbow. Orthopedic Clinics of North America 1999; 30: 15-20.

Daniels J, Zook E, Lynch J. Hand and wrist injuries: Part I. Nonemergent evaluation. American Family Physician 2004; 69: 1941-48.

Daniels J, Zook E, Lynch J. Hand and wrist injuries: Part II. Emergent evaluation. American Family Physician 2004; 69: 1949-56.

Deyo R, Rainville J, Kent D. What can the history and physical examination tell us about low back pain? JAMA 1992; 268: 760-5.

Dickey P. Surgical management of disc disease of the lumbar spine. Resident and Staff Physician 1997; 43: 41-50.

El-Gabalawy HS, Duray P, Goldbach-Mansky R. Evaluating patients with arthritis of recent onset. JAMA 2000; 284: 2368-73.

El-Khoury G, Renfrew D. Percutaneous procedures for the diagnosis and treatment of lower back pain: Diskography, facet-joint injection, and epidural injection. American Journal of Rheumatology 1991; 157: 685-91.

Frymoyer J. Back pain and sciatica. NEJM 1988; 318: 291-300.

Felson D; Osteoarthritis of the knee. NEJM 2006 354: 841-8.

Garfin S, Herkowitz H, Mirkovic S. Spinal stenosis. The Journal of Bone and Joint Surgery 1999; 81A: 572-86.

Jackson JL, O'Malley PG, Kroenke K. Evaluation of acute knee pain in primary care. Annals of Int Med 2003; 139: 575-99.

Lonner JH. A 57-year-old man with osteoarthritis of the knee. JAMA 2003; 289: 1016-25.

Luime JJ, Verhagen AP, Miedema HS. Does this patient have an instability of the shoulder or a labrum lesion? JAMA 2004; 292:1989-99.

Netter FH. Atlas of Human Anatomy, Summit, NJ; Ciba-Geigy Corporation 1989: 395-402, 476-80.

Nicholas JA. The upper extremity in sports medicine 2nd Ed, Philadelphia; Mosby 1995: 23-76.

Rectenwald, J. Stener lesion. E-Medicine 2005 http://www.emedicine.com/orthoped/topic313.htm.

Sapira JD. The Art and Science of Bedside Diagnosis. 1st edition, Baltimore; Williams and Wilkins 1990: 415-33.

Simon RR, Koenigsknecht SJ. Emergency Orthopedics, The Extremities, 3rd Ed, Stamford CT; Appleton and Lange 1996: 386-410, 437-60.

Skolnick AA. For some injuries, it's all in the name. JAMA 1998; 279: 572-73.

Smith CC. Evaluating the painful knee: A hands-on approach to acute ligamentous and meniscal injuries. Advanced Studies In Medicine 2004; 4: 362-69.

Snider RK. Essential of muscoskeletal care, 1st Ed. American Academy of Orthopedics 1997: 75-81, 311-9.

Solomon DH, Simel DL, Bates DW. Does this patient have a torn meniscus or ligament of the knee? JAMA 2001; 286: 1610-20.

Spiegel TM, Crues JV. The painful Shoulder: Diagnosis and treatment. Primary Care 1988; 15: 709-24.

Stener B. Displacement of the ruptured ulnar collateral ligament of the metarcarpo-phalangeal joint of the thumb. Journal of Bone and Joint Surgery 1962; 44b: 869-79.

Woodward TW, Best TM. The painful shoulder: Part I clinical evaluation. American Family Physician 2000; 61: 3079-88.

Sandler G. The importance of the history in the medical clinic and the cost of unnecessary tests. American Heart Journal 1980; 100: 928-31.

Bickerstaff ER. Neurological Exam in Clinical Practice. 4th edition, London; Blackwell Scientific Publications 1980.

Bickley LS. Bates' Guide to Physical Examination and History Taking. 7th edition, Philadelphia; Lippincott 1999.

Braunwalk E, Fauci A. Harrison's Principles of Internal Medicine. 15th edition, San Francisco; McGraw Hill 2001: 111-163, 2369-2441.

Caputo GM, Cavanagh PR. Assessment and management of foot disease in patients with diabetes. NEJM 1994; 331: 854-60.

Chiles BW, Cooper PR. Acute spinal injury. NEJM 1996; 334: 514-20.

Clark CM, Lee A. Prevention and treatment of the complications of diabetes mellitus. NEJM 1995; 332: 1210-17.

Cornbluth D. Peripheral neuropathy. NEJM 1982; 307: 1457.

D'Arcy C, McGee S. The Rational Clinical Examination: Does This Patient Have Carpal Tunnel Syndrome? JAMA 2000; 283: 3110-3117.

Dawson DM. Current concepts: Entrapment neuropathies of the upper extremities. NEJM 1993; 329: 2013-18.

Deyo R, Weinstein J. Low back pain. NEJM 2005; 344: 363-70.

Dyck PJ. Current concepts in neurology. The causes, classification and treatment of peripheral neuropathy. NEJM 1982; 307: 283-86.

Furman JM, Cass SP. Primary care: Benign paroxysmal positional vertigo. NEJM 1999; 341: 1590-96.

Glick TH. Neurologic Skills: Examination and Diagnosis. Boston; Blackwell Scientific Publications 1993.

Gorson KC. Case 9-2001 - A 64 year old woman with peripheral neurophathy, paraproteinemia and lymphadenopathy. NEJM 2001; 344: 917-23.

Haerer AF. Dejong's: The Neurologic Examination. 5th Edition, New York; J B Lippincott; 1992.

Hotson JR, Baloh RW. Acute vestibular syndrome. NEJM 1998; 339: 680-85.

Katz JN, Simmons BP. Carpal tunnel syndrome. NEJM 2005; 346: 1807-11.

Lange AE, Lozano AM. Parkinson's disease - First of two parts. NEJM 1998; 339: 1044-53.

Lessell S. Optic neuropathies. NEJM 1978; 299: 533-36.

Louis ED. Essential tremor. NEJM 2001; 345: 887-91.

Mancall E. Alpers and Mancall's Essentials of the Neurologic Examination. edition 2, Philadelphia; FA Davis Co; 1981.

Nathan DM. Medical progress: Long term complications of diabetes mellitus. NEJM 1993; 328: 1676-85.

Kassirer JP. Diagnostic Reasoning. Ann Intern Med 1989; 110: 893-900.

Sackett DL, Richardson WS, Rosenberg W, Haynes RB. Evidence-based Medicine: How to Practice and Teach EBM. 1st edition, Edinburgh; Churchill Livingstone 1998.

Wernick R, Coyle C. Systemic lupus erythematosus: A streamlined, rational approach to diagnosis. Hospital Medicine April 1999; 16-22.

Bowen J. Educational strategies to promote clinical diagnostic reasoning. NEJM 2006; 355 (21): 2217-25.

HOW TO CONTRIBUTE TO THIS BOOK

Please send all of your comments, edits, suggestions and reviews to:

JUDEEZEKAKPU2021@GMAIL.COM

www.ingramcontent.com/pod-product-compliance
Lightning Source LLC
LaVergne TN
LVRC080205220926
848482LV00007B/339

* 9 7 8 1 9 5 6 4 6 9 7 4 5 *